the Life Force diet

3 WEEKS TO SUPERCHARGE YOUR HEALTH AND GET SLIM WITH ENZYME-RICH FOODS

MICHELLE SCHOFFRO COOK
DNM, DAc, CNC

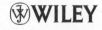

WILEY

John Wiley & Sons Canada, Ltd.

Library and Archives Canada Cataloguing in Publication Data
Cook, Michelle Schoffro
        The life force diet : supercharge your health and stay slim with enzyme-rich foods / Michelle Schoffro Cook.

Includes index.
ISBN: 978-0-470-15757-2

        1. Reducing diets. 2. Enzymes—Therapeutic use. I. Title.
RM222.2.C6578 2008   613.2'5   C2008-905758-9

Production Credits
Cover design: Frederick Evans and Anna Davidson
Interior text design: Pat Loi
Typesetter: Pat Loi
Photographer: Henrique Gendre
Printer: Friesens Printers Ltd.

John Wiley & Sons Canada, Ltd.
6045 Freemont Blvd.
Mississauga, Ontario
L5R 4J3

This book is printed with biodegradable vegetable-based inks on 55-lb. recycled cream paper, 100% post-consumer waste.

Printed in Canada

1 2 3 4 5 FP 12 11 10 09 08

Table of Contents

Luscious Life Force Recipes

Introduction

I started researching the healing power of foods 20 years ago. I had just finished reading *Fit for Life*, an excellent book that transformed my thinking about food, my body, health, and life in general. It resonated with a deep part of my being that believed that food was not meant to come in cans, contain artificial ingredients, nor be heavily processed. I started taking greater notice of the rainbow-coloured array of delicious foods that nature had bestowed upon us. I believed and continue to believe that nature holds the secrets of great health, vitality, and longevity, and that living in harmony with nature offered humanity the greatest opportunity for health and happiness.

While reading this profound book, I remember having those "aha" moments where things just make sense. Not only did I immediately change my diet, but within a few years I found myself enrolled in a holistic nutrition program—the study of how food affects us on a physical, mental, emotional, and spiritual level. I began to realize that food is not just something with which to stuff our faces, satisfy our hunger, or eat for taste alone. I learned that food was meant to satisfy our body's need for strong and healthy cells, which make up strong and healthy organs, which further organize to make up strong and healthy organ systems, and—you can guess—result in a strong and healthy human being.

My passion for natural healing was sparked and I began studying every health book I could get my hands on. I was a sponge for knowledge about the human body and natural medicines. My many book cabinets still bulge at the seams in an effort to satisfy my voracious thirst for knowledge about health and healing.

The body is absolutely miraculous: It coordinates billions of functions every second. It has the incredible ability to heal wounds, fight infection, and repair broken bones. At the smallest level, it is composed of billions of cells, millions of which are eliminated, replaced, or repaired daily. The skin is totally renewed every 28 days. The heart has replaced all its cells in only 30 days, while our lungs are completely regenerated after only 70 days! This is astounding! What's more, almost all of these functions continue to hum along quietly in the background with very little awareness from us: Our bodies have their own innate healing capacity.

After reading about the human body's extraordinary ability to heal itself, I began to wonder: If the body replaces all the cells in an organ as important as the heart in a month, why are people suffering from heart disease or other heart problems? Or, if the lungs are renewed in just over two months, why are people suffering from respiratory disorders?

While there are many possible factors that prevent health or healing, I hypothesized that *we* must be doing things that interfere with the body's innate intelligence, or that we are not giving our bodies what they need for a more complete healing. I became completely absorbed by trying to determine what things we might be doing to interfere with healing along with discovering the substances that our bodies require for healing.

I spent every spare moment researching to understand the specific conditions we must create to experience optimum health. This is a totally different perspective than the medical approach, which has minimal, if any, emphasis on factors for health and prevention of disease, but is almost exclusively focused on disease. For example, when someone suffers from the symptoms of a disease, he or she typically visits a medical doctor for a diagnosis. For the sake of example, let's say that Jane Doe is given a diagnosis of asthma. She has trouble breathing and regularly has wheezing attacks that make it almost impossible to breathe. Her medical doctor conducts an examination, reviews her symptoms, diagnoses asthma, and offers her a prescription for an inhaler to use when she feels like her airways are constricted, and a second inhaler to reduce inflammation in her airways.

The diagnosis, "asthma," from the Greek word *aazein,* simply means "sharp breath." Typically, in asthma, the airways become constricted, inflamed, and lined with mucus. But the diagnosis of asthma does not offer a clue as to why the airways are constricted and inflamed, or why there is so much mucus present in them in the first place. The medications may help open the airways but they do not address the actual factors causing the constriction, inflammation, or mucus build-up. This approach is entirely disease-focused and, while certainly valuable, offers minimal assistance in helping to heal the body from this affliction and even less insight as to the cause or causes of the disease.

If you're skeptical about whether modern medicine, as we've come to call it, is actually disease-focused, ask any medical doctor how many healthy people arrive at his or her practice looking for insight into how to maintain health. Very few—if any.

I strongly believe that modern medicine, also commonly known as "drug-based medicine," has value in its ability to minimize or eliminate disease symptoms, but little value in maintaining or creating health. Instead, I feel that nature has provided what we need to support our health, including foods and plants that have the ability to restore health. This is why I have focused my research on the latter.

Virtually every function in the human body relies on substances called enzymes to ensure that the function occurs smoothly and without any glitches. If even a single enzyme is deficient or missing, any number of serious health complications can result, depending on the specific enzyme in question. Conversely, with plentiful amounts of enzymes, the body can repair damage, slow the rate of aging, and even overcome illness.

As you will learn throughout *The Life Force Diet*, your diet holds the potential to provide the greatest source of enzymes to replenish your body's stores. I say "potential" because it requires eating a diet that contains them in the first place—something that the average person does in only minor amounts. But increasing enzyme-rich foods is easy to do and well worth the effort, as you will soon find.

Once I discovered the healing power of enzyme-rich foods, I was astounded at the health improvements I witnessed, in myself and in my clients. People dropped excessive weight; overcame colitis, irritable bowel syndrome, arthritis, fibromyalgia, and many other illnesses; and experienced an increase in energy and vitality.

I decided that I must share this exciting healing knowledge, and that is how *The Life Force Diet* came to be. I have ensured the information is easily accessible to everyone, and the program itself is easy to follow, full of delicious foods, and totally manageable for life.

The Life Force Diet is not a diet as we've come to refer to "diets." We need to reclaim the word "diet" from the clutches of weight-loss organizations that have wrongly led us to believe that "diet" is the equivalent of meagre portions, rubbery food, and deprivation. In *The Life Force Diet*, "diet" refers to a healthy way of eating for life; it refers to the other, more important senses of the word. According to *The Free Dictionary*, the other meanings of diet include: "the usual food and drink of a person or animal"; and "something used, enjoyed, or provided regularly."[1] And this is exactly what *The Life Force Diet* is all about. It is intended to be your usual food and drink, in lieu of the over-processed, overly artificial, and overly fatty nature of the average person's diet. Unlike those programs espoused in diet books that are simply not sustainable, *The Life Force Diet* is designed for lifelong health. Also unlike other programs, it is designed to be full of delicious food! Once you've experienced the delicious recipes and amazing health benefits, I am confident that you will want to enjoy it regularly throughout your lifetime—without deprivation!

You'll savour delicious soups, stews, and smoothies. You'll never eat another salad of starchy tomatoes and iceberg lettuce once you've learned how to make salads that even a salad-hater will love. And, don't think you'll be sacrificing when it comes to your sweet tooth.

Throughout *The Life Force Diet* you will be introduced to a new way of thinking about food as a living source to ramp up your life force (I'll explain more about this in the next chapter), not simply to satisfy hunger or cravings.

I'm excited to share with you information that I know will change your life … and your life force! You'll discover why we need life force foods now more than ever, and why more than 90 percent of foods we eat have little or no life force within them! No wonder so many people are exhausted and experiencing disease in record numbers.

You'll learn about the miraculous substances in our bodies and food called "enzymes," and why they're of vital importance to our well-being and our life, and why we need them to help us build a powerful life force.

Don't worry about radical changes. I'll gradually walk you through the key steps to transform even the poorest of diets into the life force diet. I'll teach you easy ways to lessen your junk food dependency, enjoy healthier versions of your favourite foods, and curb cravings. Cravings are your body's way of letting you know that you're missing key nutrients in your diet. That's why you'll never eliminate cravings on the nutrient-depleted diets most people eat. On the life force diet, however, cravings are fulfilled by the nutrient-rich and delicious foods you'll be eating.

I'll explain the powerful life force gold and silver foods you'll want to add to your diet. And, of course, I'll show you how easy it is to eat more of these delicious and satisfying foods.

Perhaps you are experiencing aches and pains, battling allergies or digestive discomfort, or experiencing a serious health condition. You'll discover how to apply the life force diet for maximum healing power. You'll learn about the incredible power of life force foods so you can stop worrying about the staggering incidence of heart disease, cancer, diabetes, and other tragic diseases and start enjoying great health.

Later in the book, I'll teach you on how to equip your kitchen for the best results, which low-cost tools are essential and which ones are just helpful additions. I'll even share helpful hints for following the diet while on the road, as well as suggestions for families, athletes, and anyone leading a busy life. You'll be amazed at how simple, inexpensive, and rewarding life force eating can be.

Feel free to flip ahead to the recipe section at the back of the book to start enjoying life force recipes immediately. You'll love Peach Pineapple Ice Cream, Plumpaya Pudding, Grilled Salmon with Salsa Violetta, and dozens of other delicious and sometimes decadent—life force foods!

In *The Life Force Diet*, you have an ally in disease prevention, healing, and unlocking the immunity, energy, and vitality that you are destined to experience. We have all heard the expression "knowledge is power." Armed with the knowledge presented in these pages, I want you to feel empowered to take an immensely important step on your journey in life. I'm honoured to take this next step toward greater life force with you!

PART**ONE**

Building Life Force
from the Inside Out

1

Your Miraculous Body

*"It's only when you're flying above it that
you realize how incredible the Earth is."*

—Philippe Perrin

IN ancient times writing was regarded as magical because it empowered the word to travel through, and even defeat, time. It is my hope
that in sharing with you the years of research and information I have
collected, you will not only turn back time within the cells of your
body and appear years younger, but revitalize the life force within
you. By replenishing your life force you will regain youthful energy
and vitality to ward off illness, embrace life to its fullest, and fulfill
your potential. In essence, you will be defeating time.

When it comes to your body, knowledge truly is power. Armed
with some inside information about what goes on in your body,
along with simple ways you can support these functions, you'll
be well on your way to great health for life. That's because you'll be
addressing your body's actual needs, not just trying to eliminate a
symptom like pharmaceutical drugs do.

What's more, unlike books or health programs that are designed
either to help you lose weight or fight disease, *The Life Force Diet* is

designed to restore balance in your body. When you do that, excess weight melts off and symptoms of ill health disappear. Your body will be healing itself from the inside ... and that's where the best and most permanent results occur. Forget diet books that don't support your health; it's time for a new way of thinking about your body and its exceptional healing capabilities.

Let's begin by taking a brief tour of the miraculous human body so you'll better understand its remarkable capacity for health and healing.

A Brief Tour of Your Miraculous Body

We don't typically give much thought to our incredible bodies until something goes wrong. Most of the time, we tend to neglect our body and not have much gratitude or appreciation for what it is doing to keep us alive. One of the things I have come to appreciate in my two decades of research into natural ways to heal the human body is that it is a marvellous creation capable of miracles. Every single second, miracles occur in your body! Millions of them! It's time we developed a new appreciation and understanding of the bodies we inhabit. Once you understand the miracle that is your body, you'll understand how great health is not only possible, but that your body is conspiring to make you feel great every minute of every day. Let's begin our journey.

Your body is one of the most extraordinary creations on the planet. While no one knows for sure the exact number of cells it comprises, scientists estimate that at the time you were born your body held about 10,000 trillion cells. That's a mind-boggling number that most of us can barely fathom. That number actually decreases as you mature and develop, and by the time you are a fully grown adult your body contains between 50 and 100 trillion cells.

About 10 percent of these cells make up the solid parts of your body such as bones, muscles, and organs. Forty percent of the cells make up the non-solid parts such as blood and lymphatic fluid. The lymphatic fluid and the network of nodes, vessels, ducts, and glands that make up the lymphatic system is the body's equivalent of a mini street-cleaning system. It transports toxins and waste products from your tissues so they can be removed from your body. It also functions as part of your immune system.

You may be shocked to learn that the remaining half of your cells are bacterial, most of which are beneficial to your body and inhabit your digestive system. An additional 100 trillion micro-organisms inhabit our ears, nose, throat, mouth, skin, and other parts of our bodies. It sounds frightening, but most of them serve important roles in helping us to stay healthy. So try not to fret that your body is home to many micro-organisms. Most of them are striving to keep you healthy and play an integral role to the vital functioning of your body. You simply could not live without them.

Each of the trillions of cells in your body is so tiny that, by some estimates, you could fit 64,000 red blood cells on the head of a pin.[1] It's hard to imagine anything so small, yet each of these cells comes complete with over a dozen structures inside itself and more on the surface. Plus, countless molecules move in and out of each cell every second.

In his book, *A Short History of Nearly Everything*, science writer Bill Bryson describes the activity within a single cell:

> If you could visit a cell you wouldn't like it. Blown up to the scale at which atoms were about the size of peas, a cell itself would be a sphere roughly half a mile across, and supported by a complex framework of girders called the cytoskeleton. Within it, millions upon millions of objects—some the size of basketballs, others the size of cars—would whiz around like bullets. There wouldn't be a place you could stand without being pummeled...thousands of times every second from every direction.[2]

·Every cell is sophisticated, and perfectly designed to perform its particular function. There are about 200 different types of cells, each of them handling a different role within your body, including breaking down food, executing genetic instructions, manufacturing chemicals and hormones needed by your body, and many others. The authors of the book *Decoding the Human Body-Field* so eloquently refer to the unimaginable speed at which everything occurs in each one of our cells as "the speed of life."[3] Every second millions of cells die and new ones are born to replace the worn-out ones.

The authors of this fascinating book also share their description of the processes within your body:

> There are millions of…activities taking place in your body during the time frames that make seconds feel like forever. In your kidneys, specialized cells are monitoring your salt and water levels, secreting hormones, and removing wastes. Amino acids are arranging themselves into strings that are making up the particular proteins that the body needs at specific times and in exact quantities. The proteins then fold themselves into the intricate three-dimensional structures that determine their function. Each configuration gives a protein a different identity, but somehow proteins know which shape to assume. Ribonucleic acid (RNA) is zipping apart the double helix of [your] DNA, copying the millions of "letters" of the genetic code, proofreading the replication and correcting any mistakes before zipping new strands of DNA back together again. Messenger RNA is receiving messages from DNA and shuttling those messages around to direct the production of enzymes and other molecules. Your heart is pumping more than a liter of blood a minute. T-cells and other immune cells are tagging, attacking, and destroying foreign organisms such as bacteria and viruses, while leaving harmless microorganisms

alone. Adenosine triphosphate (ATP), arguably the busiest molecule in the body, is being broken down to provide energy to power your cells…Thousands upon thousands of other activities and millions upon millions of chemical reactions that are absolutely crucial to your health—and to your life—are going on below the level of your awareness every minute of every day.[4]

Not only does your body organize all of these functions, it has an innate healing intelligence enabling it to mend broken bones, kill viruses, heal wounds, and much more. At any given time your body is manufacturing and using 50,000 proteins, billions of neurons are firing in your brain and nervous system, and billions of white blood cells are destroying damaging micro-organisms. And it all happens without any conscious thought from you. When people fall ill they claim to need a miracle. Typically they await a miracle drug. But in Chinese Medicine they say, "You *are* a miracle!"[5]

Yet most of us don't think too highly of our bodies, particularly if they are causing us pain or breaking down in any way. And with the exception of some degradation over time, we tend to think that our bodies are fairly unchanging: for example, your skin is the same as the skin you had last month, right? Wrong. According to experts your skin is totally renewed every 28 days. Okay, well surely the bones we had as children are more or less the same as the ones we currently have—outside of being larger and maybe a bit depleted of bone mass—but more or less they're the same, right? Wrong. Experts now estimate that all of your bone cells are totally renewed in only 90 days. But your heart must be the same heart that you had last month, last year, or at least the same as the one you were born with, right? Wrong again. Experts now tell us that every cell of your heart is entirely new in 30 days. Even complex organs such as your lungs are regenerated in only 70 days. According to quantum biologist Deepak

Chopra, in only one year your body is 98 percent renewed.[6] That means 98 percent of the body you had last year has been replaced with an entirely new one! Miraculous!

So why don't we feel like a totally new person in only a year? Well, to perform the billions of processes occurring every single second in your body, you need to ensure that your body has all the tools and raw materials it needs. Just as to change a tire on your vehicle you need a jack and a few other essential tools, or to build a home you need appropriate construction materials, your body needs the proper tools and building blocks to function properly.

Can you imagine what your home would look like if you tried to construct it out of rotted wood, frayed electrical wires, broken bricks, and leaky pipes? Not only would it look terrible, it would probably flood, crumble, or burn down. In short, it would be a health hazard. Yet this is exactly what we do with our bodies. We give them substandard fuel with which to make new cells, which then form damaged tissues or defective organs, and we're left wondering why our bodies fail us. If you treat your body well and give it what it needs, it will take care of you.

You're probably wondering what exactly your body needs to help you feel full of energy and to look and feel your best. In the next two chapters I'll share the exciting information that can help your body create a vibrant you.

2

The Building Blocks of Great Health

*"Let him who would rule the
world first rule himself."*

—Socrates

MOST of us realize that we need food and water to stay alive. We know that we cannot survive long without either of these essential items, yet we fail to consider the significant role they play in ensuring the *quality* of our life. Conversely, what happens if we fail to provide our body with high-quality food and adequate, pure water and instead attempt to nourish our body with junk food, chemical-laden food, altered fats and proteins, or other "plastic food" as I like to call it?

When I tell people that what they eat on a daily basis plays a significant role in determining the health of every cell, tissue, organ, and organ system and to their overall health, most people are shocked. But it's true. Your body becomes what you put into it. The average person wants to have their cake, donuts, steak, coffee, and perfect health too. Unfortunately, as you will soon learn, that is almost impossible. Some people eating these items on a regular basis may claim to have perfect health, but they may be experiencing only a lack of *symptoms*. Most of us know someone who eats junk food regularly, smokes like a chimney, and drinks excessively, and never seems to suffer from even a headache or stomach ache. Never, that is, until he or she suffers a heart attack or other serious ailment.

Symptoms, while uncomfortable or even downright painful, are actually positive signs: Your body is trying to communicate with you that something is wrong. Symptoms are your body's way of sending you messages that it is time to make changes in support of health. Yet most people want to eliminate them immediately with little thought as to their significance. Instead, they view uncomfortable symptoms as evidence that their body is warring against them. But it couldn't be further from the truth. In reality, your body is doing the best it can with the limited building blocks it has been given. It is essential that you give your body the best quality of building blocks to build healthy cells and tissues if you want to enjoy great health. So what exactly are these critical building blocks?

Your body has many specific needs: oxygen, water, vitamins, minerals, amino acids, fatty acids, carbohydrates, enzymes, a proper pH balance (learn more about this topic in my book *The Ultimate pH Solution*), healthy digestion and elimination, electrically charged cells, healthy emotions, love, a sense of purpose and fulfillment, and other factors for its health. If these elements are missing, your body will begin to break down and, over time, disease may be the result. Your body is not trying to make you suffer. It performs its many miraculous functions to keep you healthy, alive, and well. It simply does the best it can with the raw materials and tools you provide.

In this chapter we'll discuss the basic nutritional needs of your body. In the next chapter we'll explore the role of enzymes, which are special types of proteins that are needed to perform almost every cellular function in your body, ranging from digestion to metabolism.

Every organ, gland, and tissue in your body needs particular elements, nutrients, and other nutritional factors for optimal health. Food, air, and water provide these elements and nutrients, but when it comes to food, your body must be able to break it down into basic building blocks that can be used to build healthy cells, tissues, glands, and organs. Soon you will understand why your food choices are more capable of determining the quality of life and your body's ability to resist illness or fend off disease than any drug. But I'm getting ahead of myself. Let's explore some of the key nutritional elements needed to build a human body.

The type and quality of foods you eat (and digest, as you'll learn more about in the next chapter) determine your health or lack thereof.

Critical Elements

While there are many elements in your body, about 99 percent of the molecules in your body are formed from oxygen, carbon, hydrogen, nitrogen, and sulphur. You may recall learning about these elements on the periodic table from grade 10 science class. Don't worry, I'm not going to drag you back through high school chemistry here, but I want to give you a basic understanding of some of the critical elements your body must have for optimal functioning. I believe a better understanding of your body's needs helps you to make better food and lifestyle choices. It always astounds me when people say that their eating habits have no impact on whether they're suffering from arthritis, heart disease, fibromyalgia, cancer, or some other disease, when what they eat is one of the greatest factors for why they are suffering from illness. By understanding more about how the body functions, how it strives to heal, and how it constantly strives to renew itself, you'll understand why what you put into your body determines whether you are healthy or sick, fatigued or energized, prematurely aging or retaining your youthful looks and vigour.

You obtain the key elements I mentioned through breathing, as in the case of oxygen; drinking water, as in the case of oxygen and water; and eating nutritious foods, as in the case of the others.

The importance of breathing deeply and of obtaining fresh, oxygen-rich air cannot be overstated. Through breathing, you are helping to ensure that all the cells of your body will have the oxygen they require to perform their tasks, that is, if you inhale deeply enough and take in enough fresh air, without excessive pollutants.

Your body also needs adequate water. Water is necessary to form blood, lymph fluid, and bodily secretions, to name a few. Water also helps prevent inflammation—research now shows that inflammation is a precursor to many chronic illnesses. Water helps substances flow in and out of cells by ensuring the correct pressure between the cell and the fluid it is bathed in. It moistens the surfaces of the lungs to allow proper oxygen intake and carbon dioxide expulsion. It helps to eliminate toxins and helps remove wastes from your body. Water ensures the proper conductivity of electrical messages between brain and nerve cells. That's right, your brain and nervous system communicate via electrical messages. If you think of how lakes or rivers conduct electricity when lightning strikes, you'll have a good idea of water's essential nature in conducting electricity in your body. Water is also required for countless chemical processes in your body, along with regulating your body temperature. Without adequate water, many of your body's processes simply will not work properly.

The following table outlines some of the most common symptoms, signs, and lifestyle factors that may indicate insufficient water consumption.

Do You Need More Water?
Alcohol consumption—2 or more glasses per day
Chapped lips
Coffee or tea consumption—3 or more cups per day
Constipation (fewer than 3 bowel movements daily)
Dry mouth, eyes, or nasal membranes
Dry skin
Frequent urinary tract infections

Hemorrhoids
Small amounts of urine or urinating fewer than 6 times daily
Kidney stones
Tendency to be shocked by static electricity

Keep in mind that many of the symptoms noted as possible nutrient or water deficiency signs can also be signs of illness. You should always consult your physician to rule out any serious disease. However, it is my hypothesis that nutritional, water, or enzyme deficiencies are at the root of or a contributing factor to almost every illness, including genetic ones!

Food and Genetic Diseases

This may shock most people, but there is a whole new field of study called nutrigenomics that explores the way food and nutrition affect our genetic material. The body's production of new DNA is dependent on the presence of many vitamins. Activity of DNA is also influenced by the presence or absence of key nutrients and how they interact with genetically determined biochemical processes.

Consider the genetic disease called homocystinuria, a serious illness that affects the muscles, nervous system, connective tissue, and cardiovascular system. Scientists know it is caused by a single defective gene that triggers the release of a chemical in the body that further produces another toxic chemical called homocysteine. Although this disease is rooted in a defective gene, studies have shown that vitamin B6 in high doses can ameliorate this disease. In Jack Challem's book *Feed Your Genes*, Kilmer S. McCully, M.D., indicates that the normal activity of the chemical that triggers the production of homocysteine relies on the presence of adequate amounts of vitamin B6.[1]

Nutrients play many roles and their role as cofactors with our genes is one of their most significant. As Jack Challem clearly states in the same book, "Nutrients provide the building blocks of genes and they turn many genes on and off. Because you control what you put into your mouth you can literally feed your genes right and gain tremendous health benefits."[2]

He also recounts learning about a physician who used large dosages of vitamins and other nutritional supplements to treat children with Down's syndrome, a disorder caused by a genetic defect that leads to physical and mental disabilities. The earlier the physician treated these children, the more likely they would experience near normal intelligence and appearance as they matured. Researchers have also known for decades that inadequate amounts of folic acid, a B-complex vitamin found in leafy greens, during pregnancy can increase the risk of the birth defect spina bifida in children.

Your genes coordinate the creation of everything in your body ranging from your physical features (such as hair or skin colour) to the inner functioning of bodily processes. But even your genes depend on the avoidance of substances that cause genetic damage like smoking and ingesting certain food additives (we'll discuss this topic in more detail in Chapter 4), and the proper intake of nutrients found in food to do their work.

The Nutrients in Food

Nutrients are classified as either macronutrients or micronutrients based on the amounts typically required by our bodies. Macronutrients include amino acids, sugars, and fatty acids, which are cellular building blocks found in proteins, carbohydrates, and fats, respectively. In other words, your body breaks down protein into amino acids, carbohydrates into sugars, and fats into fatty acids for its needs—that is, if the food you eat contains quality sources of these nutrients and if your body is capable of properly digesting the foods and extracting these macronutrients. We'll be talking about excellent sources of these nutrients and ways to improve your body's ability to extract these nutrients throughout *The Life Force Diet*.

Protein Power?

After water, proteins make up the bulk of our body weight. Once a protein food is ingested, the digestive system breaks it down into its amino acid constituents. Then our DNA instructs our body as to how to put these amino acids back together, depending on our body's specific needs. Our bodies need a range of the 20 different amino acids found in protein-rich foods to make up the many different protein chains that form our muscles, blood, skin, hair, nails, and internal organs such as the brain and heart. Even our genetic material is made up of chains of amino acids. From amino acids, our bodies make chemical messengers called neurotransmitters that allow our brain to communicate with our body, as well as other hormones to regulate our emotional activity. The hormones that control many functions such as growth, sexual development, and metabolism are also created from amino acids.

While most people assume that the only (and therefore, best) source of protein is meat, that is incorrect. Although animal protein and fish certainly are sources of protein, they are definitely not the only ones. There are many excellent vegetarian sources of protein, including lentils; soy products; black beans, aduki, and other beans; walnuts, almonds, and other nuts; sunflower seeds; pumpkin seeds; sesame seeds; brown rice; and other whole grains. Even vegetables and fruits contain some protein. Actually, an avocado contains more useable protein than an 8-ounce steak—not to mention many healthy fats, fibre, and other nutrients!

While amino acid deficiencies may be the result of consuming insufficient protein in underprivileged nations, this is rarely the case in Western cultures. More often, amino acid deficiencies are the result of poor digestion or inadequate variety of protein sources. We'll be discussing many ways you can improve your digestion in the coming chapters. Most people notice dramatic digestion improvements on *The Life Force Diet*.

There are many symptoms and signs that you may be deficient in amino acids found in protein. Following is a chart to help you understand whether you may be deficient. Keep in mind that this list is not exhaustive, nor does it mean that you are definitely deficient if you have one or more of these symptoms.

Symptoms of an Amino Acid Deficiency
"Hang nails" or cuticles that tear easily
Addictions (cigarettes, alcohol, sugar, caffeine, work, etc.)
Anemia
Anxiety or anxiety attacks
Bloodshot eyes
Brittle or cracked nails
Cataracts
Chronic fatigue
Cold sores, herpes simplex
Depression
Difficulty concentrating
Difficulty handling stress
Dry hair, split ends, or hair falling out
Excessive appetite
Forgetfulness
Frequent colds, flu, or other infections
Hair loss
Headaches or migraines
Heart disease (diagnosed by a doctor, also called cardiovascular disease)
High blood pressure
High triglycerides (based on blood tests)

Hyperactivity
Insomnia
Irritability
Lack of coordination
Loss of muscle mass
Lupus erythematosus
Mood swings
Muscle weakness

Carbs, Carbs, and More Carbs

We hear so much about "low-carb" foods and diets that you would think all carbohydrates are poison, but that's far from the truth. In reality, you couldn't live without carbohydrates. The problem is that most people choose the wrong kinds of carbs. There are two kinds of carbohydrates: complex and simple. Complex carbohydrates are healthy carbohydrates found in whole grains, vegetables, and some fruit, whereas simple carbs are foods that contain glucose, fructose (fruit sugar), or milk sugar. Here are some examples of foods that are simple carbohydrates: cakes, cookies, pastries, ice cream, and many so-called fruit juices. They are found in most prepared and fast foods, including store-bought salad dressings and condiments. In fact, most people are suffering the ravages of sugar overload—partially the result of these carbs, which are also linked to disease and premature aging.

I have not included a chart of carbohydrate deficiency symptoms because it is almost unheard of. Conversely, as you will learn in Chapter 4, most people eat excessive amounts of the wrong types of carbohydrates and are experiencing the resulting blood sugar fluctuations, weight gain, and mood swings that are linked to excessive or poor carb choices.

Fibre is actually a type of carbohydrate. However, in our bodies it tends to function differently. Instead of providing energy in the form of glucose, fibre's role is to protect the health of the intestinal tract by adding bulk to the stools, which decreases transit time of waste matter in the intestines and thereby lessens the likelihood that toxic, microbial, or carcinogenic wastes can absorb into the blood, and consequently lessens the risk of intestinal disorders.

While experts suggest that the body needs between 35 and 40 grams of fibre daily, most people ingest only about 20 grams. So it's not a surprise that they are also experiencing chronic constipation and the resulting toxicity. Fibre is divided into two types: soluble and insoluble. Soluble fibre is a gummy substance that is found in grains, seeds, and legumes, as well as in the edible parts of vegetables and fruits. Soluble fibre can help lower cholesterol in the body by binding to it and escorting it out. Insoluble fibre is also found in many grains, nuts, seeds, vegetables, and fruits, but does not break down. It helps to ensure that the intestines maintain their shape and lessen the likelihood of irritable bowel syndrome.

Other than poor food choices, the primary reason people don't eat adequate amounts of fibre is that they are concerned about experiencing gas. As complex carbohydrates (fibre included) are digested by bacteria in the intestines, gas is released. However, you can easily avoid this problem by eating smaller amounts of fibrous foods more frequently throughout the day. Unless you are making a substantial effort to eat at least 35 grams of fibre, you are most likely not getting enough fibre in your diet. Following is a chart of some of the common ailments and symptoms linked to inadequate fibre consumption.

Symptoms of a Fibre Deficiency
Abdominal bloating
Constipated (fewer than 3 bowel movements daily)
Hemorrhoids
Overweight or obese
Painful bowel movements
Small appetite
Suffer from or have suffered from gallstones
Varicose veins

Essential Fatty Acids

Essential fatty acids are obtained through eating foods such as avocados, flaxseeds, olive oil, wild salmon, nuts, and seeds. There are many different types of fatty acids, including linoleic acid (LA) or Omega 6s, alpha linolenic acid (ALA), eicosapentanoic acid (EPA), and docosahexanoic acid (DHA). ALA, EPA, and DHA are various types of Omega 3 fatty acids. Both LA and ALA are found in many types of nuts, seeds, leafy greens, and other vegetarian sources, while EPA and DHA are found in fish or fish oil supplements.

Don't worry. You don't have to memorize their names or acronyms to benefit from the various types of essential fatty acids. What's most important is that you understand their purpose in your diet and how to balance the ratio of the different types.

Essential fatty acids perform many functions in our bodies, including quelling inflammation, strengthening and supporting the adrenal and thyroid glands, protecting nerves and the brain, maintaining healthy heart and arterial function, and maintaining healthy skin and a healthy hormonal balance.

Most cells in the body use essential fatty acids to ensure proper fluidity. For example, most people eat excessive amounts of harmful saturated fats found in meat. This high level of saturated fat combined with our typically low levels of essential fatty acids can result in cells that are excessively fluid,[3] and may be more vulnerable to damaging toxins in the body. The brain is approximately 60 percent fat and needs essential fatty acids to ensure proper brain health. Brain and nerve cells require proper cellular fluidity to function properly. Changes in cellular fluidity of these cells can affect behaviour, mood, and even mental functioning.[4]

If your diet contains trans fats, the harmful chemically altered fats found in many types of margarine, baked goods, prepared and fast foods, then you need to know that not only do these fats replace beneficial ones needed for the healthy functioning of your body, but they may cause serious damage (you'll learn more about these fats in Chapter 4).

There are many symptoms and signs that you may be deficient in one or more essential fatty acid. Following is a chart to help you understand whether you may be deficient. Keep in mind that this list is not exhaustive, nor does it mean that you are definitely deficient if you have one or more of these symptoms.

Symptoms of an Essential Fatty Acid Deficiency
Acne
Arthritis
Asthma
Attention deficit disorder or short attention span
Bleeding gums or tendency to bruise easily
Brittle or cracked nails
Depression
Diabetes
Dry eyes or tear ducts
Dry hair, split ends, or abnormal hair loss
Dry mouth or throat, especially when speaking
Dry or scaly skin
Eczema, psoriasis, or dermatitis
Forgetfulness
Frequent colds, flu, or other infections
Irritability
Overweight or obesity
Slow-healing wounds or injuries
Women: PMS (Premenstrual syndrome) or difficulty getting pregnant or carrying to full term

Vitamins

On the micronutrient level, your body requires vitamins and minerals. The exact amounts required by your body are most likely different from anyone else on the planet, but we all need many different vitamins and minerals in sufficient quantities for our bodies to function properly.

Let's take a brief look at some of the vitamins and minerals needed by your body, the functions they perform, and some of the signs of deficiencies.

Vitamins have diverse roles in our body, including functioning as hormones in the case of vitamin D, or as antioxidants that protect against free radical damage as in the case of what I call the "ACE vitamins" or vitamins A, C, and E. Some vitamins assist with the signalling and regulation of cell and tissue growth, while others are precursors of critical enzymes in our body (more on enzymes in the next chapter). Other vitamins act as transport shuttles between enzymes to carry certain chemicals needed to function properly.

Without adequate vitamins and minerals in your diet, your body will not be able to support healthy bone, eye, gland, skin, teeth, hair, heart, lungs, hormonal, brain, and nervous system functioning, among others.

I'll share a quick overview of some of the individual vitamins your body needs and what roles they play in your body.

Vitamin A

Vitamin A helps ensure healthy eyes, hair, and bones; maintains strong adrenal glands; and is critical to a healthy immune system. Your nails, hair, skin, and teeth all require vitamin A to grow or function properly. Vitamin A, or its precursor, beta carotene, is found in yellow-orange fruits and vegetables like carrots, squash, melon, papaya, and mango, as well as dark leafy greens and fish oils.

Symptoms of a Vitamin A Deficiency
Acne or blackheads
Cysts or boils in ears or mouth
Dry eyes

Continued on page 28

Continued from page 27

Symptoms of a Vitamin A Deficiency
Dry hair, split ends, or hair falling out
Dry or scaly skin
Dry, scaly, or red eyelids
Eye inflammation or pink eye (conjunctivitis)
Eyes have difficulty adjusting when entering a dark room
Eyes sensitive to sunlight, glare, or bright lights
Frequent colds, flu, or other infections
Reduced night vision or inability to see in dim light
Rough bumps on the back of arms
Sinus problems or sinusitis
Swollen eyelids or sties on eyelids
Urinary tract infections (also bladder or kidney infections, also called cystitis)
Warts

B Vitamins

There are many vitamins found within the B-complex, including B1, B2, niacin, pantothenic acid, B6, folic acid, B12, B13, B15, B17, choline, inositol, biotin, and PABA. It's not necessary to remember all of these vitamins. It's just important to recognize that they play a critical role in many of our bodily functions. Our glands require one or more of the B-complex vitamins to manufacture proper hormones, which can play a role in many of our emotions. Without adequate quantities we become more susceptible to stress, depression, anxiety, or irritability. B-complex vitamins are necessary for adequate energy, learning capacity, growth, immunity, reproduction, pain reduction or proper pain signals, wound healing, memory, and glandular and nervous system functions. For many of my clients, I start by increasing their consumption of foods rich in B-complex vitamins such as brown rice, root vegetables, pumpkin seeds, citrus fruits, strawberries, cantaloupe, kale, green vegetables, and beans, and they soon start to feel more energetic and more capable of handling their lives, as well as having more balanced moods.

Symptoms of a B-Complex Vitamin Deficiency
Anemia, fatigue, or weakness
Anxiety, irritability, or nervousness
Cold sores or canker sores in mouth
Depression, anxiety, or irritability
Dizzy or lightheaded when standing up
Dry hair, split ends, or abnormal hair loss
Fleeting pains or tenderness in joints or legs
Forgetfulness or short attention span
Frequent colds, flu, or other infections
Hang nails or cuticles that tear easily
Headaches
Heart palpitations or slow or rapid heartbeat
High blood pressure
Insomnia or difficulty staying asleep
Irregular heartbeat
Lack of endurance or fatigue easily
Muscle cramps in legs, especially after exercising
Prematurely aging skin or wrinkling
Rapid heartbeat with slightest exertion
Restless leg syndrome
Shortness of breath or chest pains
Skin bruises easily
Skin is itchy, red, or inflamed (dermatitis)
Weight loss or loss of appetite
White skin patches
Women: Acne or swelling is worse during periods, menstrual problems, morning sickness during pregnancy

Vitamin C

While most people know that vitamin C is important to help ward off cold and flu viruses, few people are aware that this crucial vitamin plays an important role in bone and tooth formation, digestion, and blood cell formation. It helps accelerate wound healing, produces collagen which helps maintain skin's youthful elasticity, and is essential to helping us cope with stress. It even appears to help protect our body against toxins that may be linked to cancer. Our stress glands, the adrenal glands, which are two small, triangular-shaped glands that sit atop the kidneys in the abdominal area, use a large amount of vitamin C. That means the more stress we're experiencing, the more vitamin C our bodies deplete. Alcohol consumption and cigarette smoking also quickly deplete vitamin C in our body. Because vitamin C is water soluble, it is not stored in our body and must therefore be ingested on a regular basis to avoid a deficiency. There are many vitamin C deficiency symptoms. The following chart is a sampling of some of the most common ones. Some of the foods that have high amounts of vitamin C include oranges, lemons, grapefruit, limes, pomegranates, strawberries, black currants, spinach, beet greens, tomatoes, many types of sprouts, and red peppers.

Symptoms of a Vitamin C Deficiency
Anemia
Excessive hair loss
Exhaust easily
Fragile bones
Frequent nosebleeds
Gums bleed easily, especially when brushing or flossing teeth
Premature aging of skin
Prone to catching cold, flu, or other infections easily
Skin bruises easily
Sores, wounds, or infections that heal slowly

Vitamin D

Vitamin D is considered both a vitamin and a hormone, since it has hormonal effects in our bodies. It is primarily made in our bodies as a result of getting adequate sunlight. You may have heard about seasonal affective disorder (or SAD, as it is also called), which is linked to inadequate sunlight and therefore a vitamin D deficiency. Vitamin D plays an important role in our energy levels, moods, and helps to build healthy bones, heart, nerves, skin, and teeth, and it supports the thyroid gland. While sunlight is the primary source of this important vitamin, it is also found in fish and fish oil, sweet potatoes, sunflower seeds, mushrooms, and in many types of sprouts.

Symptoms of a Vitamin D Deficiency
Bow legs or knock knees (rickets)
Burning in mouth or throat
Constipation
Dental cavities or cracked teeth
Insomnia
Joint pains or bone pains
Muscle cramps
Nearsightedness or myopia (can't see distances)
Nervousness
Osteomalacia
Osteoporosis
Poor bone development

Vitamin E

Vitamin E is an important antioxidant vitamin. As a result, it plays an important role in combating the effects of aging. Without adequate vitamin E, your body's blood vessels, heart, liver, lungs, adrenal and pituitary glands, skin, testes or uterus, and other important tissues would suffer. Vitamin E helps protect your body from toxins in the environment and your food. It is found in many whole grains and whole grain breads, cereals, and sprouts, as well as dark leafy vegetables, nuts, and seeds.

Symptoms of a Vitamin E Deficiency
Anemia
Blood clots or tendency to form blood clots
Celiac disease
Cystic fibrosis
Dry hair, split ends, or hair falling out
Eye twitching
Men: impotence or low sex drive
Muscle weakness or swelling or loss of muscle mass
Poor coordination
Women: menstrual pain

Minerals

You now understand the important role of many of the key vitamins found in foods. Minerals also play a critical role in your health, not the least of which involves their ability to function as coenzymes to ensure that enzymes are manufactured and perform their thousands of vital roles in every aspect of the biochemistry of your body.[5] There are dozens of minerals: Let's explore some of the main ones.

Calcium

Most people think "bones" when they think of calcium. Calcium is arguably involved in more biological functions than any other mineral. From bone health to muscle movement to our beating heart, calcium is critical on the cellular level. Yet calcium is one of the most misunderstood minerals. While it is found in high amounts in dairy products, you'll learn in the coming chapters why these foods are not the best sources and why, even if you eat plentiful amounts of dairy products, your body may not be extracting enough calcium for its needs. Unfortunately, while Americans and Canadians eat among the highest amount of dairy products in the world per capita, we are still suffering from many calcium deficiency symptoms and disorders. Calcium also plays an important role in building and maintaining strong teeth, nails, blood, skin, and soft tissues. It is essential to our brain's ability to connect with our body via proper nerve signals. Additionally, it helps relax our nerves, helping us to cope with stress. It's no coincidence that we are eating calcium-deficient diets and most people are highly "stressed out." Excellent and highly useable sources of calcium include carrot juice, kale, dark leafy greens, sesame seeds and tahini (sesame butter), broccoli, almonds and almond butter, kelp, oats, and navy beans.

Symptoms of a Calcium Deficiency
Back or hip pain
Bone loss, malformed bones, or bones that are vulnerable to fractures or breaks
Brittle nails or vertical ridges on nails
Cramps in feet, toes, or legs
Dental cavities or frequent toothaches
Headaches
Heart palpitations
High blood pressure
Insomnia
Joint pain
Muscle twitching
Nervous tics or twitches
Nervousness, anxiety, or irritability
Women: painful or lengthy periods or excessive bleeding during periods

Chromium

Chromium, while an important mineral, is often overlooked. It helps maintain strong arteries, blood, and heart health, and it also plays a significant role in alleviating a "sweet tooth." Chromium lessens cravings, mood swings, and weight gain linked to fluctuating blood sugar levels since it helps to keep them balanced. Chromium also plays an important role in energy production in our bodies. Interestingly, chromium is naturally found in sugar cane, which makes sense: It would effectively help our bodies handle the high sugar content of this food. However, industry removes all of this mineral and many others to create what we've come to know as white sugar (which, I'd add, now has no value in our diet). Chromium is also naturally found in many grains, beans, and potatoes.

Symptoms of a Chromium Deficiency
Cravings for sugary or starchy foods
Diabetes or hypoglycemia (or chronically high or low blood sugar)
Difficulty tolerating alcohol or sugar
High cholesterol
High triglycerides

Iodine

Not just found in table salt, iodine is imperative to the proper functioning of the thyroid gland—a butterfly-shaped gland in the throat that helps with metabolism, energy, moods, and temperature regulation in our body. Like chromium, iodine assists with energy production and metabolism. Iodine is also important to regulate the function of the nervous system and brain, and helps to support healthy hair, nails, skin, and teeth. While most table salt has been iodized, I do not recommend obtaining iodine by using table salt, since it is devoid of most other minerals and, of course, is loaded with sodium. Many types of seaweed contain the highest concentrations of iodine, including kelp, dulse, arame, wakame, agar, etc. Garlic, watercress, summer squash, sesame seeds, pineapples, pears, peaches, pumpkins, and moderate use of Himalayan crystal or Celtic sea salt are also good sources of iodine.

Symptoms of an Iodine Deficiency
Brittle nails
Cold hands and/or feet
Constipation
Dry hair
Heart palpitations
High cholesterol levels
Irritability
Overweight or obesity
Slow mental reactions
Slow metabolism
Thyroid enlargement or goitre
Women: fibrocystic breasts or breast lumps

Iron

Most people are aware that we need the mineral iron to have adequate energy, but iron plays other important roles in our body, including red and white blood cell production, resistance to stress, proper immune functioning, and the metabolizing of protein, among other things. Iron is also a key constituent of enzymes within immune system cells that attack foreign invaders such as bacteria, fungi, and viruses to neutralize them before they can cause disease in your body. Most nutritionists explain that there are two types of iron, heme and non-heme, and advise people that heme iron from meat sources is best absorbed by the body. While that is partly true, most red meat sources of iron contain excessive hormones, antibiotics, saturated fats, and other substances that negate much of the value of the iron they contain. Vegetarian (non-heme) sources of iron include prunes, raisins, figs, apricots, bananas, walnuts, kelp, beans, lentils, dark leafy greens, asparagus, and peaches. Incidentally, most of these foods also contain vitamin C, which helps with the absorption of iron in the body.

Symptoms of an Iron Deficiency
Breathing difficulties
Brittle or soft nails or vertical ridges on nails
Chronic fatigue
Cravings for ice or tendency to eat ice
Intolerance to cold
Lack of stamina or endurance
Nails are flat or concave (curved in like spoons)
Pale fingernails
Pale inner skin on lower eyelid
Pale skin
Poor attention span
Weakened immune system

Magnesium

Magnesium is the partner mineral to calcium. Typically wherever calcium is needed in the body, magnesium is also required. Magnesium is the relaxation and anti-stress mineral, since it plays an important role in helping our bodies combat stress. It is necessary for healthy artery, blood, bone, heart, muscle, and nerve function, yet experts estimate that approximately 80 percent of the population in North America may be deficient in this important mineral. Magnesium is vitally important to our health and well-being. It is involved in the production of energy for most of our bodily processes and even the structuring of our basic genetic material is dependent on adequate amounts of magnesium. Your body also requires adequate supplies of magnesium to manufacture the approximately 500 enzymes needed for basic life and metabolic functions. Magnesium is found in almonds, sesame seeds, sunflower seeds, almonds, figs, lemons, apples, dark leafy greens, celery, alfalfa sprouts, brown rice, and many other sources.

Symptoms of a Magnesium Deficiency
Back pain
Carpal tunnel syndrome
Chronic fatigue
Confusion
Cravings for chocolate
Depression
Dizziness
Epilepsy or convulsions
Excessive body odour
Heart palpitations or irregular heartbeat
High blood pressure
Hyperactivity or restlessness
Inability to control bladder
Insomnia
Irritability or anxiety
Muscle cramps or muscle tension
Nervous tics or twitches, or muscles that twitch or spasm
Pain in knees or hips
Painful and cold feet or hands
Restless legs especially at night
Seizures, convulsions, or tremors
Sensitive or loose teeth
Women: PMS or painful periods

Potassium

One of the important electrolytes that help regulate heartbeat and nerve signals is potassium. Like the other electrolytes (calcium, magnesium, and sodium), potassium performs many essential functions, some of which include relaxing muscle contractions and converting glucose into fuel that can be stored for later use by our body, reducing swelling, and protecting and controling the activity of the kidneys, body fluids, and acid/alkaline balance. For more information about the importance of the latter, see my book *The Ultimate pH Solution*. Without adequate potassium in your diet, your body cannot preserve the maximum health of your blood, heart, kidneys, muscles, nerves, and skin. Bananas are a well-known and good source of potassium. Other valuable sources of this mineral include most vegetables (particularly dark green leafy ones), citrus fruits, apricots, tomatoes, sunflower seeds, whole grains, and potatoes.

Symptoms of a Potassium Deficiency
Constipation
Dry skin
Extreme thirst
Fluid retention in hands or ankles
Heart palpitations, irregular heartbeat, slow or rapid heartbeat
High blood pressure
Irritability or easily agitated
Muscular weakness
Painful or abnormally stiff muscles after exercising

Silica

Silica, or silicon as it is also known, plays an important role in building strong bones, strengthening your immune system against invaders; assisting in the proper use of calcium in your body; and encouraging strong hair, nails, and teeth. It also supports the formation of an important enzyme called prolyhydroxylase in your body, which is involved with the formation of collagen in bones, cartilage, and connective tissue. Silica is found in flaxseeds, oats, whole grains, almonds, sunflower seeds, celery, apples, strawberries, grapes, kelp, onion, parsnips, and beets.

Symptoms of a Silica Deficiency
Excessive wrinkling of the skin
Insomnia
Irritability
Muscle cramps
Poor bone development
Soft or brittle nails
Thinning or loss of hair

Zinc

One of the most critical nutrients needed for burn and wound healing of all kinds, zinc also encourages proper digestion and utilization of carbohydrate foods like grains, vegetables, fruits, and sugars, and protein foods like meat, eggs, and beans. Men typically have high zinc needs to support healthy prostate function. Zinc helps to ensure healthy reproductive organ growth and development and maturity. Zinc is necessary for the body to manufacture at least 200 different enzymes needed for various aspects of metabolism and life. Our blood, bones, brain, heart, liver, and muscles also depend on adequate levels of this important mineral to function healthily. Zinc is found in many types of sprouts, pumpkin seeds, onions, sunflower seeds, nuts, dark leafy green vegetables, beets or beet greens, carrots, and peas, among other foods.

Symptoms of a Zinc Deficiency
Acne
Anorexia or small appetite
Brittle nails
Children/teenagers: growing pains, stunted growth
Diarrhea
Difficulty conceiving children
Frequent colds, flu, or infections
Hair or nails grow slowly

Continued on page 40

Continued from page 39

Symptoms of a Zinc Deficiency
Loss of sense of smell or taste
Men: late sexual maturity, prostate disorders, impotence, or low sperm count
Sleep disturbances
Slow hair or nail growth
Slow-healing wounds or injuries
Stretch marks
White spots on fingernails

While there are many other vitamins and minerals that play important roles in our body, the ones above are some of the most crucial ones. As you can see, vitamins and minerals perform diverse and essential roles, and without adequate amounts of these important nutrients, our bodies simply do not have adequate building blocks of healthy cells, tissues, organs, and organ systems. When we have insufficient vitamins and minerals, we will fail to experience the vitality and life force intended for us. But vitamins and minerals are not the only nutritional factors we need to consider for optimum health. Our bodies also require a healthy balance of probiotics in our intestinal tract and enzymes in our foods. I'll discuss the latter in great detail in the next chapter, but first let's take a quick look at the role of probiotics.

Probiotics and the Role of Bacteria

In Chapter 1, you discovered that approximately half of your body's cells are bacteria and that an additional 100 trillion bacteria inhabit various parts of your body and play critical roles in your health. You could not survive without these micro-organisms. Probiotics are a group of micro-organisms that play an essential role in ensuring the proper elimination of waste materials from the intestines, manufacturing of important nutrients, controlling harmful bacteria and yeast populations like candida, and other necessary functions.

There are over 150 species of harmful yeasts known as candida, but the one that frequently becomes overgrown in our intestines is *Candida albicans*. The overgrowth of this yeast causes a common condition known as *candidiasis*. While it is rarely diagnosed by medical doctors who often fail to recognize the commonplace occurrence and the harmful nature of the condition, candidiasis can cause many negative health effects. Some of the symptoms include allergic reactions, environmental or food sensitivities, acne, eczema, rashes, hives, attention deficit disorder (ADD) or attention deficit and hyperactivity disorder (ADHD), bloating, anxiety, PMS, insomnia, joint and muscle aches, among many others.

Probiotics, the beneficial bacteria, help to keep candida in check. More recently, research is showing that these "friendly bacteria," as they are sometimes called, play a critical role in brain health as well (for more information, consult my book *The Brain Wash*). I've included a chart of signs or symptoms that may indicate that you have insufficient probiotics in your intestines to help keep harmful bacteria and yeasts at bay and perform other health-promoting functions.

Common Signs You May Have Insufficient Probiotic Bacteria in Your Body
Acne
Bloating
Bruise easily
Cold sores, canker sores, or herpes simplex
Constipation
Diarrhea
Eczema or psoriasis
Heart disease
Hemorrhoids
High cholesterol

Continued on page 42

Continued from page 41

Common Signs You May Have Insufficient Probiotic Bacteria in Your Body
Indigestion
Intestinal gas
Irritable bowel syndrome
Nosebleeds
Urinary tract infections (also bladder or kidney infections, also called cystitis)
Yeast infections or candida overgrowth

The Foods We Eat

The central tenet of *The Life Force Diet* is that the foods we eat need to replenish our vitality and life force. These foods build healthy cells that further build healthy bodies, as well as tasting great, and they are not just be a means of satisfying hunger or cravings. When I was creating the life force diet as a way to restore my own health and vitality that had been faltering, I first considered the many principles I had learned about how the body functions best, which foods support health and life, which ones interfere with bodily processes, and how to employ those foods that have the greatest healing ability to restore our bodies to optimal performance on every level—starting from the cells through to tissues and organ systems. The result: life force foods.

As you'll soon learn, life force foods are the secret weapon against aging, excess weight, and disease of all kinds. In addition to the many vitamins, minerals, natural plant pigments, and other healing phyto-nutrients found in life force foods, many life force foods are packed with miracle healing substances called enzymes. Enzymes in foods were only discovered over the past several decades, yet are showing tremendous promise to prevent or heal disease, restore great health, slow the aging process, and help with weight loss. They are incredibly powerful and wide-acting because they help restore the function of our natural bodily processes and biochemical functions. In other words, they don't just eliminate symptoms: They get to the root cause of our suffering. But I'm getting ahead of myself. I'll explain more about enzymes, what they are, and their miraculous healing abilities in the next chapter.

3

Explore the Miracle
Healing Power of Enzymes

*"To become different from what we are, we
must have some awareness of what we are."*

—Bruce Lee

IN some cultures language is more than a way of communicating; it is an expression of the most important components of daily life. For example, every symbol of the ancient Norse alphabet represented a particular aspect of primeval life. A particular S-like letter resembled a lightning strike and represented both the sun's energy and the spark of energy that they recognized as existing within all living beings. They treated both the sun's energy and the human life force energy as sacred.

Life force can be measured in the electromagnetic field that our bodies transmit, or understood to be a more etheric form of energy that science is only in the early stages of discovering and understanding. Most of us are aware that we are more than just a collection of bones, muscles, cells, and other physical forms. While these bodily parts are important, as are the many biochemical processes that occur within our bodies, we are not simply the sum of these parts and processes.

Indeed, there is a spark that initiates and organizes processes within our body to keep us alive, functioning, and healthy.

We can easily support or diminish this spark through our lifestyle and food choices, and nutrition plays a massive role in keeping the spark strong. However, our typical modern diet is not designed to help us stay strong and vital: It is not supporting our life force.

If you are like most people, you are probably deficient in at least one important dietary factor that is leaving you tired, overweight, and at risk for many major illnesses and weakening your life force. Researchers estimate that 80 percent of women may be suffering from an overlooked deficiency. I suspect it is in the same vicinity for men and that this estimate may actually be low. And I'm not talking about a deficiency in protein, calcium, vitamins, or essential fatty acids—important nutrients that we discussed in the last chapter. This deficiency is even more widespread than most of the common nutrient deficiencies we hear about, yet virtually no one in the medical community knows about this potentially serious epidemic. The missing nutritional factor I'm talking about is enzymes.

Throughout history and the world, the curative properties of foods, particularly enzyme-rich foods, have been known. In the early 1900s a man named Dr. Szekely translated books entitled the *Essene Gospel of Peace, Books I–IV*, authored by a Jewish sect called the Essenes, who lived between 200 and 300 BC. According to his translation, this group of people ate grains that they sprouted and dried in the sun. This gospel is one of the earliest references to an enzyme-rich diet. Going back even further, scientific evidence has shown that early humans ate an enzyme-rich, largely plant-based diet for millennia.

I am not suggesting that we revert to the dietary habits of our ancient ancestors, but neither should we discard these habits in favour of "modern" processed foods devoid of nutrition and life-supporting capacity. By simply making better food and lifestyle choices we can build a strong life force, vibrant energy, and potent immunity against disease, thereby enabling us to live life to its fullest.

Let's begin our exploration of enzymes that can help us increase our lifespan and maximize our health. Research by one of the earliest enzymologists, Dr. Edward Howell, revealed that enzyme shortages are commonly seen in people suffering from chronic diseases, including allergies, premature aging, some forms of cancer, heart disease, skin conditions, and obesity.[1]

Enzymes are used in vast quantities in our bodies to quell inflammation, promote wound healing, and regenerate tissues, all of which are essential processes to handle most chronic illnesses. So it should come as no surprise that illness and injury may deplete our body's enzyme manufacturing abilities. To counter this depletion we need to ingest more enzymes through food and supplementation (more on the latter later in this book). Dr. Howell described the balance between the need for enzymes, the depletion of enzymes, and the replenishing of enzymes through food as our "enzyme account." Like bank accounts, if we always withdraw and never make deposits, we will eventually deplete our resources.

An interesting study conducted by Francis Pottenger Jr., MD, in his report entitled "Pottenger's Cats," demonstrates the damage that can occur by depleting our enzyme accounts—even over multiple generations! He conducted a decade-long study of 600 cats, feeding them a diet of food completely devoid of enzymes. The first generation of cats started suffering from "heart problems; nearsightedness, farsightedness; under activity of the thyroid or inflammation of the thyroid gland; infection of the kidney, of the liver, of the testes, of the ovaries; arthritis, inflammation of the joints; inflammation of the nervous system with paralysis and meningitis."[2]

The next generation of cats had symptoms worse than their parents. Pottenger found that they were "much more irritable, dangerous to handle, sex interest is slack or perverted, role reversal, allergies, and skin lesions."[3] While about 25 percent of the cats born to the first generation died, Pottenger noted that 70 percent of the cats born to the second generation died. The deliveries were more difficult and more of the pregnant cats died in labour.

The third generation of kittens suffered from similar health conditions. None lived past six months and, as a result, they were unable to produce offspring. There was no fourth generation.

For comparison, Pottenger fed another group of cats an enzyme-rich diet of raw meat, raw milk, and cod liver oil, since cats are carnivorous animals. He observed healthy cats from one generation to the next. As an interesting footnote to this experiment, Dr. Pottenger also studied the plants that he fertilized from the cats' manure. The plants fertilized by the manure of the cats that ate the enzyme-rich diet grew well, while the plants fertilized by the manure of the cats that ate the enzyme-deficient diet were also weak and struggled to survive. The lack of life force enzymes had ramifications that were multi-generational and even affected other species.

Pottenger's study certainly notes the importance of enzyme-rich food in the diets of cats. Not surprisingly, the newest research is showing the importance of an enzyme-rich diet for humans as well.

Doctor Hans Eppinger, chief medical doctor at the First Medical Clinic of the University of Vienna, conducted research into the effects of eating an enzyme-rich diet. He found that enzyme-rich foods significantly improved the ability of the cells to be selective, that is, to eliminate toxins and absorb nutrients.

Additionally, he was aware that our cells conduct electricity and that a drop in the cell's electrical potential is the first step in the disease process—even before laboratory and diagnostic tests indicate disease. After testing numerous types of foods, he and his colleagues found that enzyme-rich foods were the only ones that could restore the electrical potential in weak or damaged tissues.[4] This exciting research shows the curative potential of enzyme-rich foods.

Do you know that humans are the only animal to drink the milk of another species? We're also the only species that cooks and processes its food (although we also process and cook the food for animals we've domesticated, and incidentally they have many of the same diseases from which we suffer). When I think of the severe negative impact on the cats after only three generations of eating exclusively cooked foods without enzymes, I am concerned about the consequences for humans of the foods we consume. Three generations ago, the quantity of junk food, processed food, and food additives was considerably lower than it is today. Arguably, the quality and quantity of enzyme-rich fruits and vegetables in the daily diet was also greater three generations ago. What will our children and our children's children be facing as generational and genetic damage from low- or no-enzyme diets has an impact on their health?

Enzyme Miracles

Dr. Wolfgang Bringmann and Dr. Rudolf Kunze, of Berlin, Germany, conducted a study of athletes at an official mini marathon. For two days prior to the event Dr. Bringmann gave the athletes 10 enzyme tablets three times per day. On the morning of the event, the athletes took 10 additional enzyme supplements. The athletes maintained their strict training schedules throughout this test. Dr. Kunze took blood samples of the athletes and observed that the levels of lymphocytes, a substance created by the body as part of an immune system response typically indicating physical stress, were remarkably reduced, which indicated that the athletes' bodies were less stressed by their physical activity.

Dr. Anthony Cichoke cites exciting information about the effects of enzymes on rheumatoid arthritis in his book *Enzymes & Enzyme Therapy*. He indicates that rheumatoid arthritis improves or is at least delayed when high doses of enzymes are used over an extended period of time.[5]

Other research shows the tremendous promise enzymes offer to sufferers of HIV (human immunodeficiency virus). An estimated 33.2 million people are currently suffering from HIV, including the 1.3 million sufferers of this tragic disease in North America.[6] According to research in Germany and Puerto Rico, the use of enzymes to treat these illnesses is having positive results.[7]

While multinational pharmaceutical giants continue to search for a synthetic chemical to cure disease (to the tune of trillions of dollars, I might add), miraculous healing enzymes that have the power to heal disease and restore health exist in a banquet of Mother Nature's foods and in enzyme supplements extracted from foods.

The Spark

When I talk about enzymes, most people gaze at me with a confused expression and an uncertainty as to whether they've ever even heard of enzymes. At the beginning of the chapter I referred to a "spark"—an action that helps our body do the important things it needs to do not only to be healthy, but to keep us alive. Enzymes are sparks. Without a spark, we could not start a vehicle, create a fire for warmth, or even light a candle. The spark begins the process of creating fire—a process we've learned to harness for many of our modern needs.

Our bodies rely on a spark that, like the spark creating fire, initiates thousands of biochemical processes. Our bodies rely on enzymes to ensure all of the many internal biochemical functions are initiated and maintained. Just by their existence they ensure that all of the processes within our 100 trillion cells occur smoothly. Without them our bodies' essential functions would break down and disease would result. Enzymes are critical to life. Without enzymes, almost nothing would happen in your body. Without adequate amounts in your diet, you may be vulnerable to weight gain, bloating, fatigue, asthma, arthritis, high cholesterol, pain, and countless other health concerns.

Unlike vitamins and minerals, enzymes are not considered nutrients—instead, they are catalysts, meaning that they act like brokers, linking two compounds to ensure they react with each other. Meanwhile the enzyme remains unchanged.

Each enzyme has a particular function. One enzyme cannot and does not do the work of another enzyme. For example, a specific enzyme can link the nutrient folic acid (vitamin B9) with cholesterol that's stuck in an artery wall, allowing the folic acid to begin to dissolve the blockage. No other enzyme can fulfil this role. However, without this critical enzyme the folic acid could not perform *its* vital function.

Clearly then, enzymes play crucial roles in keeping our bodies healthy. Enzymes can combine with close to 100,000 compounds, including many of the nutrients we discussed in the previous chapter. These compounds are called cofactors, and together they trigger a multitude of actions. Almost nothing can happen in your body without the assistance of enzymes.

While solid research has been available to the medical community for almost a century, it has been largely ignored. Even today, most of the information taught about enzymes in schools is outdated. Let's take a look at the fundamentals of enzymes.

Enzymes 101

Enzymes are a special type of protein that is necessary for every chemical reaction in your body, including the normal functioning of cells, fluids, tissues, organs, and organ systems. **Enzymes are uniquely different from other protein molecules because they are biologically active.** In other words, they contain life force energy.

Types of Enzymes

There are currently over 5000 known enzymes and some experts anticipate that there are at least as many still waiting to be discovered.

But they all fall into three main categories: digestive, metabolic, and plant enzymes. Let's explore these kinds of enzymes.

Digestive Enzymes

Digestive enzymes assist with breaking down foods into their nutrient components for proper absorption. They are also called pancreatic enzymes, since they are primarily secreted by the pancreas, an organ found just under the lower left side of your rib cage. The pancreas regulates blood sugar levels through the production and secretion of a hormone called insulin. It also manufactures and secretes over 20 enzymes that are essential to digestion, including amylase, lipase, and protease enzymes. These enzymes digest carbohydrates, fats, and proteins respectively.

Metabolic Enzymes

Metabolic enzymes are made by the body to properly run all of its biochemical processes, from moving and talking, to breathing and thinking. Each one of these enzymes has a unique function for which it is created. If any particular metabolic enzyme is missing or deficient in the body, it can lead to any number of serious diseases.

One particular type of enzyme that you may have heard about is a group called antioxidant enzymes. Different from antioxidant nutrients like vitamin C and E that we must ingest to benefit from their antioxidant effects, antioxidant enzymes are a type of metabolic enzyme that is manufactured inside our bodies for the specific purpose of destroying harmful substances called free radicals. We hear about free radicals frequently in the media as research uncovers their link to many diseases. A free radical is an atom or molecule with an unpaired electron. You may remember from science class that electrons surround the nucleus of an atom in pairs. A missing electron means the atom or molecule is more positively charged and highly reactive. In our bodies, the free radical will seek out other molecules or atoms to steal an electron, creating additional free radicals and wreaking havoc at the cellular level.

Free radicals form naturally during metabolism and our body is designed to combat them. But our exposure to free radicals is increased by our exposure to toxins and chemicals in our air, food, and water. This spawns more free radicals. When our diet is low in antioxidants such as vitamin C, which destroy free radicals, we are less capable of overcoming the excess, and our bodies must expend substantial energy in the manufacture of antioxidant enzymes in an effort to keep up with the free radicals. This is an enormous task as we are increasingly exposed to more free radicals and ingesting fewer antioxidant nutrients. If our bodies cannot keep pace with the free radicals, we sustain cellular damage, we age faster, and we are more prone to illness.

Perhaps enzymes have been overlooked by most doctors because there has been confusion about the connection between this class of enzymes—metabolic enzymes—and digestive enzymes. While they assist with different bodily functions (the latter obviously aids diges- tion), they are both produced by the same organs—the pancreas and liver. We'll learn more about these important organs momentarily. For now, it is important to understand that if our bodies don't have adequate amounts of digestive enzymes, the pancreas and liver shift their focus from creating essential metabolic enzymes to assisting with digestion. In other words, digestion of food is such a significant function in our bodies that the manufacturing of critical enzymes for other metabolic processes may fall short if the body needs help in breaking down food. That's no surprise when you recall our ear- lier discussion about the vital importance of our body's ability to break down food into the building blocks of cells, hormones, tissues, glands, and organs.

So potentially thousands of life-supporting metabolic processes, including burning fat for energy, may suffer if there is a deficiency of enzymes in the body. And, you guessed it: This enzyme deficiency is linked, at least in part, to our current obesity and overweight epidemic.

First for Women magazine conducted an interview with Joseph Brasco, MD, gastroenterologist at The Center for Colon & Digestive Diseases in Huntsville, Alabama. In the interview he discusses the way in which a lack of enzymes derived from food forces the liver and pancreas to expend their energy creating digestive enzymes for the purpose of breaking down a meal. He adds: "Because the pancreas and liver need energy to produce enzymes, the resulting drain renders these organs temporarily unable to perform their functions of detoxification, blood sugar control, and fat burning."[8] And that's just the start. The result of the impairment of just these three functions can lead us to feel exhausted, suffer from mood swings, and become overweight. Over the longer term, we become more vulnerable to chronic illness like heart disease or diabetes. And with 500 other functions to perform, the liver needs all the energy it can muster.

Plant Enzymes

Sometimes called food enzymes, plant enzymes are found in raw plants such as fruits, vegetables, and herbs. By eating a diet rich in plant enzymes, you will dramatically reduce the number of digestive enzymes your body needs to manufacture, freeing up energy and making more enzymes available to the body for healing! That's why the life force diet focuses on eating more foods with substantial amounts of plant enzymes, or life force, as it's also known. These life force rich foods not only assist with digestion, but also have enormous healing implications.

Yet due to food processing and heating techniques, enzymes are almost completely depleted from our food supply. According to prominent enzyme researcher Dr. Ellen Cutler, 70 percent of American women get almost no enzymes in their diet.[9] And, the same number likely applies to men. Actually, many men are more likely to avoid fruits and vegetables and forego responsible eating for a diet rich in enzyme-deficient cooked meat and processed fare. It makes sense that they would be also be at risk of enzyme depletion.

Eating more enzyme-rich foods like the Life Force Gold Foods I'll discuss in the coming chapters is one simple way of increasing the amount of plant enzymes in our bodies. Doing so not only improves digestion, it also helps prevent the pancreas and liver from turning their focus to digestion, better enabling them to focus on their important metabolic functions in our bodies.

Now let's discuss digestion so you'll have a better understanding as to why increasing life force enzymes can help improve your digestion, and the potentially vast implications of doing so.

A Brief Tour of Digestion

Here's a quick look at what happens when you eat something—let's take an apple. The digestive tract comprises many organs, including the mouth, tongue, stomach, small intestine, large intestine (also known as the colon), liver, gallbladder, and pancreas. While there are others, we're just looking for an overview here and don't need to delve too deeply into every organ and function.

From the moment you bite into that apple, digestion begins. While teeth are not traditionally included in the digestive system, they play an important role in digestion, by breaking food down so that other organs can better perform their functions on the food. While you're chewing your food, the salivary glands secrete juices full of amylase enzymes—three different kinds—that immediately start digesting the apple, or any other food containing carbohydrates you might eat. Not only does chewing well speed up the digestive process, it lessens the load on the organs, freeing valuable energy for other tasks, including restoring health and vitality.

You may recall that enzymes each have one function. In the case of amylase enzymes, their job is to digest all forms of carbohydrates, including fruit, sugary foods, grains, beans, and starchy vegetables. So the apple begins to break down from chewing, and enzymes secreted in your mouth as well as those released from chewing the apple start to break it down further. Chewing is actually a stage of digestion— and an immensely important one at that. Chewing liberates enzymes within the food itself (provided they were not destroyed during food preparation) and mixes the food with enzymes secreted in your saliva to partially digest the food.

After you swallow the chewed apple, it passes through a tube called the esophagus until it reaches the stomach, which is divided into two chambers. The first chamber is like a holding station where the enzymes that were secreted earlier, along with those naturally released by chewing the food, can continue working. The food sits in this chamber for half an hour to 45 minutes and then moves on to the second chamber. The second chamber secretes and bathes the food in pepsin and hydrochloric acid to break down any protein it contains. Many people are shocked to learn that apples contain protein, but this is true. Actually, all fruits and vegetables contain some protein. But the stomach works primarily on heavily concentrated proteins found in foods like chicken, beef, eggs, dairy, and other animal products. How long the food spends in the second chamber is dependent on a number of factors, including how much concentrated protein was eaten, the efficiency of your digestive system, and whether you drink any liquids while eating or soon afterward.

If you drink water, juice, coffee, tea, or another beverage just prior to eating, while eating, or within an hour or so of eating, you'll dilute the body's digestive enzymes, especially the hydrochloric acid in the stomach, making it less capable of digesting the food and prematurely signalling to the intestines that the stomach's job is done, even if it isn't. So it's important not to drink with meals; otherwise, you'll weaken digestion. And as you'll soon learn, strong digestion is critical to the health of just about every function in the body.

Once the food leaves the stomach, or typically after it has been in the lower chamber of the stomach for about two hours or longer, it (combined with pepsin and hydrochloric acid) is passed down to the approximately 23-foot-long small intestines. Already a fluid-type substance, it mixes with additional fluids produced by the liver, pancreas, and small intestines. The body completes a sort of nutritional inventory to determine which enzymes are required to complete the digestion process.[10] The liver, a large and powerful organ located just beneath your ribs on the right side of your body, produces a green-coloured fluid called bile that the gallbladder stores and secretes as needed to assist with digestion, especially of the fats found in foods. The pancreas, a skinny organ that sits beneath the stomach on the left side to the middle of your abdomen, secretes fluid that contains bicarbonate (a substance similar to baking soda) that helps neutralize acid from the stomach, along with several enzymes, including amylase, chymotrypsin, lipase, trypsin, and others, all of which further digest the food. You may recall that we mentioned amylase and lipase earlier, as they are two essential enzymes needed to digest the starchy and fatty parts of food, respectively. These and other enzymes secreted by this important organ are involved in digesting all types of foods, including carbohydrates, fats, and proteins.

The mucous membrane of the small intestines secretes additional enzymes to continue the digestion process. While the now unrecognizable apple is in the intestines, it undergoes additional digestion, remaining nutrients it contained are absorbed, and any remaining unabsorbed food passes down to the large intestines. In the small intestines, water and various nutrients are absorbed directly into the bloodstream through the intestinal walls. In addition to critical vitamins and minerals, the building blocks of carbs, fats, and proteins—sugars, fatty acids, and amino acids—are also absorbed before the remaining matter passes to the large intestines.

Once food passes through the small intestines and the water and nutrients absorbed through the walls of the intestines move into the blood, the remaining matter continues through the large intestines until it is eliminated from the body during bowel movements. Insufficient water, fibre, or enzyme-rich food can impair the process of digestion, contributing to constipation, and causing waste products to be absorbed through the intestinal walls into the blood, and ultimately to organs and tissues throughout the body. That's why it is important to have two to three substantial bowel movements daily. If you're experiencing fewer than that, or conversely, if you frequently experience diarrhea, your digestion may be not be functioning as well as it should. If your bowel movements contain undigested food particles, that may also be a sign of improper digestion.

Chew Your Food!

Mom was right when she told you to chew your food. Without adequate chewing, your body misses a whole step of digestion—and an immensely important step at that. And since every digestive organ is designed for specific purposes, they can't do each other's jobs. In other words, the stomach, intestines, or other organs simply cannot chew food. Remember that without sufficient chewing, the food will not mix with enough enzymes to break down carbohydrates, nor will the enzymes in the food be fully released, meaning that the food will miss the opportunity to break down while in the holding chamber that is the upper portion of the stomach. A semi-chewed apple would move to the stomach, but because it is a carbohydrate, the stomach has little role to play. Your body will be forced to create enzymes to break down the food, which is not sufficiently chewed, to make up for the lack of digestive enzymes usually released in the saliva through adequate chewing, and to make up for the enzymes that remain locked inside the large pieces of apple now moving through your system. And, while you can create enzymes to digest the natural sugars found in the apple, your body cannot manufacture enzymes to break down the fibre, resulting in difficulty digesting the apple, or other fruits and vegetables. If you've ever heard people say they cannot tolerate eating fruit, they probably weren't chewing their food well enough!

Let's look at other things that take place in both the small and large intestines that are critical to good health. As you know our intestines are home to many micro-organisms—actually about 100 trillion, which rivals the total number of cells in your body. Many of these healthy micro-organisms assist with proper digestion and immune functioning, and help ensure brain health. Frequently, however, the intestines can be overrun by harmful micro-organisms such as fungi called *Candida albicans*. In a healthy person, the ratio is approximately 85 percent good micro-organisms to 15 percent pathogenic ones, but in many people this ratio may tip in favour of the harmful ones, causing enzymes to be redirected to deal with the harmful overgrowth. That means that there are fewer enzymes, both those manufactured by the body and those extracted from food, to help break down food and ensure the absorption of nutrients through the intestinal walls into the blood, which is the normal channel by which nutrients are incorporated into our bodies.

Candida or other damaging micro-organisms can become overgrown due to excessive sugar, meat (particularly meat that contains antibiotics or added hormones), or processed food consumption, use of the birth control pill, alcohol intake, blood sugar imbalances, use of steroid medications like cortisone and inhalers, mercury dental amalgams, recreational drug use, stress, mold exposures, weakened immunity, or multiple sexual partners. If you think you may have a candida overgrowth, odds are you're right. Candida overgrowth is extremely common thanks to our modern diet and lifestyle habits. Eliminate sugar, meats, and processed foods and follow the life force diet and you will start to see great improvements.

Digestion—the Foundation of Great Health

We have often heard the adage, "You are what you eat." I would add to that, "You are what you eat, digest, absorb, and assimilate." Healthy digestion is critical to virtually every function in your body.

No matter what disease a person presents with in my office, I strive to improve his or her digestion. Without excellent digestion, a person simply cannot have great health. It's that simple. Yet few people give a second thought to the health of their digestion, preferring to pop an antacid to stop any suffering rather than explore how their lifestyle and nutritional habits may be at fault for their indigestion, heartburn, or gas. We cannot expect to guzzle carbonated beverages, eat meat or other animal protein at every meal, have our daily rich desserts, and still enjoy perfect digestion … or perfect health.

There are many reasons why digestion is the foundation of superb health. Let's explore them.

First, proper breakdown and absorption of nutrients are essential to every biochemical process in your body, from replenishing dead cells to eliminating inflammation and pain. As you saw with the apple example above, this is a complex process. During digestion, foods are broken down into their building blocks—water, sugars, fatty acids, and amino acids on a larger scale, and vitamins, minerals, and other nutrients on a smaller scale. Every single one of these nutrients is required for great health! Let's look at the most commonly known mineral—calcium—which is only one of dozens of minerals your body needs for health. Calcium is essential to healthy bones, teeth, nails, blood, heart, skin, and even soft tissues like muscles. If your digestion is poor, you'll fail to break down foods into their nutrient components; in this example, you would fail to absorb into your blood the calcium from foods you eat. No amount of money spent on calcium supplementation will correct the digestive problem and thereby correct the deficiency. Without addressing the digestive system first, you'll have expensive calcium-rich urine while continuing to suffer from any number of the many calcium-deficiency symptoms or signs like bone loss, heart palpitations or irregular heartbeat, sensitivity to noise, high blood pressure, anxiety, irritability, or many others. And calcium is just one of dozens of nutrients that perform important functions in the human body.

The second reason that strong digestion is essential to health is that the gastrointestinal tract, also known as the GI tract, houses an important component of the immune system. The stomach's hydrochloric acid can kill many micro-organisms that may enter our bodies through contaminated food. Mucus found in the GI tract also helps to neutralize pathogens. Additionally, enzymes in the intestines help neutralize substances that cause the immune system to overreact, including toxins from pollution.

Third, research shows a link between the health of the brain and the GI tract, often referred to as the "gut-brain connection." The gut is also called the "second brain" because it plays such a significant role in protecting the brain from disease. In other words, brain health is, at least in part, a reflection of what's happening in our digestive system. If the digestion process is impaired, your body will lack adequate building blocks to maintain healthy brain and nervous system cells. The GI tract is one of the main determinants of the levels of inflammation in your body and whether your body will attack healthy tissue, including your brain.

Fourth, beyond your brain and nervous system, a healthy digestive tract lessens inflammation that has been linked to many serious, chronic health conditions. Beneficial micro-organisms in the intestines eliminate harmful pathogens and manufacture nutrients essential for many bodily functions. If harmful micro-organisms become out of balance in the intestines, they can irritate the lining of the intestines and increase the permeability of the intestinal wall—sometimes called leaky gut syndrome—a common condition in which the intestinal walls become porous and allow wastes, toxins, harmful micro-organisms, or undigested food particles to travel through the walls and into the bloodstream. Once in the blood, the immune system may overreact to these foreign substances, which may be linked to autoimmune disorders like rheumatoid arthritis, multiple sclerosis (MS), celiac disease, and many others.

You'll learn more about the importance of digestion and what you can do to improve both your digestion and the assimilation of nutrients in your body throughout this book but the following box can help you get started immediately.

Improve Your Digestion Right Now

1. Thoroughly chew your food.
2. Don't drink any liquids half an hour before, during, or one hour after meals. If you are taking any supplements with food, limit the amount of water to ½ cup or just enough to swallow the supplements.
3. Drink lots of water throughout the rest of the day away from meals.
4. Eat lots of fibre-rich foods like beans and veggies.
5. Reduce your consumption of meat, sweets, processed foods, soft drinks, and alcohol.
6. Supplement with a full-spectrum digestive enzyme supplements. (More on this topic later in the book.)

What Do Plant Enzymes Do?

Every food in its natural uncooked state contains both the proportion and the varieties of enzymes required to digest itself, provided it is not heated above 118 degrees Fahrenheit. If you leave a bowl of fresh fruit sitting on your table and forget about it for awhile soon (perhaps go away on holiday) you'll be greeted by a bowl of rotting fruit. What's happening is that the enzymes in the fruit (potentially alongside bacteria) start to break down the fruit sugars and other components. A similar process occurs in the digestive track, except instead of days or weeks in the bowl, the digestion process takes place over hours.

All foods in their natural state contain the specific enzymes that will break them down. So foods that contain higher amounts of fat such as olives or avocados will also contain the enzymes that digest fat—lipase. Foods that are higher in carbohydrates like berries or peaches contain more of the enzymes that break down carbs—amylase.

As you discovered earlier, protein, carbohydrates, and fat are essential components of food that are necessary for many functions. Enzymes help to release their building blocks of amino acids, sugars, and fatty acids, thereby releasing the energy contained in foods for building healthy cells, tissues, organs, and organ systems.

By chewing foods replete with enzymes, we rupture the cell walls of the food, releasing these enzymes so they can begin to do their work. There are four groups of enzymes found in plant-based foods such as fruit, vegetables, beans, grains, nuts, and seeds. They include:

1. **Proteases** break down the lengthy protein molecules into smaller amino acid chains and then eventually into individual amino acids.
2. **Amylases** break down polysaccharides into disaccharides, which simply means that they turn complex carbohydrates into simple sugars. "Poly" means many, "saccharides" means sugar, and "di" means two.

3. **Lipases** break fats (called triglycerides) into individual fatty acids and a substance called glycerol. When the body burns fat for energy, it releases both fatty acids and glycerol into the bloodstream. Enzymes in the liver convert the glycol to glucose to provide energy for cellular metabolism. This is one of the essential fuels for smooth-running cells.

4. **Cellulases** specifically break apart the bonds found in plant fibre, called cellulose, to release another form of glucose to fuel the body.

Conditions for Enzymes to Work

Simply eating enzyme-rich food is not enough. Enzymes are something of nutritional prima donnas, requiring very specific conditions to do their work, or they simply won't work at all. They need a specific pH, temperature range, and moisture. Other factors such as cooking, medication, and the presence of certain heavy metals can also interfere with the ability of enzymes in your body to function properly.

pHinding Balance

If you have ever used the natural cleaning products baking soda and vinegar, you already have some insight into pH. The term "pH" stands for "potential of hydrogen," which is the measure of acidity or alkalinity on a scale of 0 to 14. Zero is the most acidic reading while 14 is the most alkaline reading. At the mid-point (7) you'll find neutral—a complete balance between acid and alkaline. Vinegar is highly acidic while baking soda is alkaline. If you've poured baking soda down a drain and added vinegar, you'll watch the two fizz. They are chemically reacting to balance each other's acidity and alkaline levels to obtain neutrality.

Most of your body, your blood included, needs to be slightly alkaline. In the blood, the ideal is 7.365 (or slightly alkaline). Due to our consumption of highly acid-forming foods like meat, poultry, dairy products, sugar, sweets, and others, our bodies have to deal with excess acid, which not only strains the detoxification mechanisms, it is a burden to the body's alkaline mineral reserves, thereby potentially weakening bones and muscles.

Enzymes in our bodies require a fairly balanced pH, erring on the side of alkalinity. If our bodies become too acidic, primarily through an acid-forming diet, chronic stress, a lack of exercise, and toxic exposures, then fewer enzymes may be manufactured by our bodies and those that are may not work properly or at all. The more acidic our bodies are, the less effective our enzyme activity. Not only does this affect digestion, it affects almost every bodily function.

Drugs and Toxins

Medications and toxins that we're exposed to in our food, air, and water supply can interfere with enzymes by throwing off our bodies' delicate pH balance, depleting critical nutrients needed as coenzymes or enzyme cofactors, or by directly inhibiting the action of enzymes. I'm not suggesting that you discontinue your medications, but be aware that you may have a greater need to eat a higher proportion of enzyme-rich foods like the Life Force Gold Foods you'll learn about momentarily. Always consult with your physician if you want to stop taking or lessen your dose of prescription medications.

The Temperature's Rising

Plant enzymes need the temperature to fall between 92 and 104 degrees Fahrenheit. In other words, body temperature provides the ideal amount of heat for enzymes to begin their work.

Enzymes found in plant foods must have moisture to function properly. Water molecules are required for enzymes to break apart molecular bonds in the food. So, in our bodies, saliva serves this purpose perfectly. Ensuring that you drink enough water throughout the day helps to provide the moisture needed for the many enzyme-mediated biochemical reactions to take place in your body.

The Toxic Hazard

Many toxins and heavy metals, once inside our bodies, can interfere with the capacity of enzymes to work. For example, the heavy metals lead and mercury bind to enzymes. Once these metals bind to an enzyme, they do one of three things to it: 1) denature the enzyme; 2) inhibit the enzyme's ability to function at all; or 3) denature and inhibit the enzyme. The result can be disastrous—degenerative diseases, nerve damage, or potentially even death.[11]

Unfortunately our exposure to toxins and heavy metals is unprecedented in our human evolution, thanks largely to the industrial revolution and our extensive use of these harmful substances in manufacturing and industry. Lead and mercury are frequently found in food, particularly junk food and packaged food, making it increasingly important to eliminate these health-destroyers from our diets (and I'll explain how in the next chapter). Lead is found in water supplies fed by lead pipes in older homes, refined chocolate, and canned food, as well as cigarette smoke, glossy and coloured newsprint, and leaded candle wicks. Mercury typically finds its way into our bodies through immunizations as a preservative or through farmed fish or fish known to contain high levels of mercury such as king mackerel, shark, swordfish, tilefish, tuna, and farmed salmon. Metal amalgam dental fillings, found in many people's teeth, contain high levels of mercury that vaporize in the presence of hot or acidic foods, which is then inhaled into the bloodstream.

In week 1 of the life force diet you'll eliminate many of these food sources of lead and mercury along with countless other toxins that really have no place in food. And if you smoke, I'm sure you don't need one more person telling you it's time to quit. But, from a toxic exposure perspective, it has never been more important than now to kick the habit. Your body deserves better treatment than your past bad habits may have offered. It's never too late to make a fresh start on quitting smoking, establishing good eating and exercise habits and a positive perspective on life.

Enzyme Potential

Enzymes are the ultimate philanthropists. They give all of their energy to perform their specific biological activity until they are completely exhausted. At that point they become like any other protein in the body and are absorbed.

The traditional school of thought on enzymes was that the body had unlimited quantities to ensure the proper functioning of every bodily process, under almost any circumstance, for as long as we lived. However, newer research indicates that we have a limited number of enzymes that must last throughout our lifetime.

Dr. Edward Howell coined the term "enzyme potential" during his many years of research on enzymes that culminated in his book *Enzyme Nutrition*. He says that our enzyme potential is the number of enzymes we have the ability to produce in our bodies during our lifetime. He proposed the concept that our lifespan was linked to our enzyme potential and that once we used up our potential to create enzymes, our lives would end. There is still debate among scientists and nutritionists as to whether this theory is accurate, but it seems fairly straightforward that the more enzymes we deplete through digestion, the less energy we have available for the remaining metabolic functions in our body.

And this sentiment is proving accurate. Roy Walfor, MD, reduced the daily food intake of mice in his laboratory at UCLA (thereby reducing the enzymes required for digesting the food) and observed that the mice lived 25 percent longer. While there are no lifelong human studies that confirm a link between reduced food intake and increased lifespan, short-term trials indicate that it is linked to reduced body weight, blood pressure, cholesterol levels, and blood glucose—all of which are risk factors for two of the major killers: heart disease and diabetes.[12]

Now, I'm not going to suggest that you substantially reduce the volume of food you ingest every day, but by increasing the food's own enzymes (and therefore life force) you will reduce the amount of enzymes your body must manufacture to digest the food, thereby achieving a similar result—operating at what is called "metabolic efficiency"—the concept Dr. Walfor proposed from the results of his study. And not only does increasing enzymes in our foods have the potential to increase our lifespan, it has the power to improve your quality of life, as you will learn momentarily.

Our Enzyme-Depleted Diet

Our so-called modern diet is replete with many weaknesses—it is high in trans fats, saturated fats, sugar, chemical food additives, sodium, and other less-than-desirables. It contains insufficient amounts of essential fatty acids, many vitamins and minerals, phytochemicals (natural healing compounds found in plant foods), and enzymes. I'll share the problems in the typical diet in the coming chapters and provide the steps we need to take to transform our diet from seriously horrendous to supremely healthy. For now, let's take a look at the reasons our food is almost totally devoid of life force.

Most enzymes are destroyed at 118 degrees Fahrenheit. No, that's not a typo and I didn't mean to state Celsius. At 118 degrees Fahrenheit, which is actually not that hot, enzymes are destroyed, rendering them incapable of digesting food and releasing the many nutrients locked inside the natural foods we eat.

Most of our food supply is cooked well beyond that temperature, ensuring that there is no life force and minimal nutritional value left by the time we sit down to eat it. If the food has been processed at all, it has been exposed to high temperatures even before we buy it. All canned, bottled, and packaged food is heated to high temperatures prior to lining grocery store shelves. Even oils like vegetable, sunflower, safflower, and canola oils have been heated to over 500 degrees Fahrenheit prior to being packaged. So, before you add a single degree of heat to your food, most of it has already been heated to the point of killing its life force.

At home, we fry, sauté, bake, broil, BBQ, microwave, or steam the food, ensuring that any life force that may be left is now gone. Cooking food will ensure that you don't get any additional enzymes and that you will kill the ones that exist in the food. I'm not suggesting that you stop cooking your food altogether. Not at all. However, there are some methods like deep frying and microwaving that I think you should eliminate from your life, since they are known to chemically alter fat and protein molecules in food, making them less recognizable or useable to your body. Other than deep frying and microwaving, I want you to understand that some cooked food in your diet can be helpful in ensuring that you obtain certain important nutrients. However, it is advisable to increase the amount of enzyme-rich, uncooked food you eat to about 50 percent of your diet. This will ensure maximum health, ideal body weight, and increase your life force energy to ward off disease. You may be having visions of rabbit food just now, but don't worry, I won't leave you eating like a rabbit. I wouldn't eat like one. I absolutely love delicious and gourmet foods, so I don't expect you to eat any differently than I would. You'll soon see that you can eat delicious food that is packed with life force enzymes. You just need to learn a few simple tricks that I'll teach you throughout the rest of this book to effortlessly maximize your life force enzymes.

Coenzyme Helpers

Whether foods are cooked or not, it is also important to eat a diet high in the nutrients we discussed in the previous chapter for all the reasons already mentioned, and also to ensure the proper functioning of our bodies' own enzymes as well. That's because many of the nutrients mentioned function as coenzymes in our bodies. Coenzymes are substances found in food that are necessary for an enzyme to function. Since our bodies cannot manufacture coenzymes, we must obtain them in our diet. Coenzymes include various nutrients such as vitamins B1 and B2, niacin, pantothenic acid, vitamin B6, folate, vitamin B12, biotin, vitamin C, and lipoic acid (also known as coenzyme Q10 or ubiquinone). Coenzymes are used up while performing their important functions in the body and enabling enzymes to work. That means that we need to replace them regularly or we'll run the risk that our bodies will have insufficient quantities to enable enzymes to function.

The first eight nutrients I mentioned here are all part of the B-complex vitamins (including niacin, pantothenic acid, folate, and biotin) so you can see how important it is to ensure that your body has enough B-complex vitamins. All nutrients that function as co-enzymes are water soluble and absorbed through the walls of the intestines, where the majority are stored in a form that is bound to enzymes. They play a critical role in a wide variety of biochemical reactions, including cellular energy production. That's part of the reason that so many people who begin to eat a diet rich in B-complex vitamins or supplement with them alongside a healthy diet notice an improvement in their energy levels.

Even if you have sufficient enzymes in your body, most of them cannot perform properly without the presence of these important nutrients on an ongoing basis. What's more, in the case of the B-complex vitamins, they are all interdependent. In other words, if you are deficient in one, you may develop deficiencies in the others as well. I've included a handy chart to help you understand the important role of the B-complex vitamins and their role of coenzymes in your body.

B-Complex Vitamins Function as Coenzymes[13]	
B-Complex Vitamin and Its Coenzyme Form	**Primary Function as a Coenzyme**
Vitamin B1 (thiamine) Thiamine pyrophosphate (TPP)	Energy creation and metabolism
Vitamin B2 (riboflavin) Flavin mononucleotide (FMN) and flavin dinucleotide (FAD)	Energy creation and metabolism
Niacin (B3) Nicotinamide adenine dinucleotide (NAD) and Nicotinamide adenine dinucleotide (NADP)	Energy creation and metabolism
Pantothenic Acid (B5) Coenzyme A and numerous other coenzymes	Energy creation and metabolism
Vitamin B6 Pyridoxal phosphate (PLP) and pyridoxamine phosphate (PMP)	Digestion and absorption of fatty acids found in fats and amino acids found in protein foods
Folate (B9) Dihydrofolate (DHF) and tetrahydrofolate (THF)	DNA synthesis
Vitamin B12 Methylcobalamin and deoxyadenosylcobalamin	New cell synthesis and the reformation of folate coenzymes in the body
Biotin Coenzyme R	· Energy creation and metabolism · Digestion and absorption of fatty acids from fats, amino acids from protein foods · Synthesis of glycogen (a form of stored energy in the body)

Some people may have noticed that the fat-soluble vitamins like vitamin A, D, E, and K are not considered coenzymes. However, they *are* critical to so many bodily functions, so it is still important to obtain them through your diet and moderate sunlight exposure in the case of vitamin D.

If your body is unable to produce sufficient quantities of pancreatic enzymes (secreted by your pancreas), then you may not absorb fat-soluble vitamins. So the importance of supporting your body's internal enzyme production through healthy nutrition also helps to ensure you can absorb the nutrients your body needs from food. It's a symbiotic relationship, and one that demonstrates the importance of getting more enzymes in your diet to lift the burden of manufacturing so many enzymes inside your body.

Consider the case of people who consume excessive alcohol over long periods of time. Excessive alcohol consumption can impair the pancreas and liver, causing insufficient enzyme and bile production respectively. Since both are needed to absorb vitamin A, for example, many alcoholics suffer from severe vitamin A deficiency and the resulting deficiency symptoms. Incidentally, alcohol consumption depletes vitamin C and the B-complex vitamins that are imperative to enzyme functions in the body.

Many prescription medications like those used in chemotherapy for cancer, diuretics, antibacterial drugs, and others also deplete the important coenzyme nutrients, rendering them incapable of performing their important enzyme assisting roles.

Coenzyme Q10, which is also known as lipoic acid or ubiquinone, is both made in our bodies and found in many foods like nuts, seeds, whole grains, and fatty fish. This nutrient is essential to almost every biochemical reaction in your body, so it is imperative that your body obtain enough of it to ensure that your cells have sufficient energy to perform their countless tasks. Otherwise, these processes can become impaired. Coenzyme Q10 is naturally found in uncooked, enzyme-rich foods, but is typically depleted in a diet consisting of processed foods. As a result, most people are likely deficient in this nutrient and coenzyme. Your body can make more, provided it has adequate amounts of the amino acids phenylalanine and tyrosine, vitamin E, and the B-complex vitamins thiamine, pyridoxine, and folate.

The scientific director at the Lupus Research Institute in Ridgefield, Connecticut, Dr. Emile Bliznakov, was able to extend the lifespan of mice through their intake of CoQ10. He divided old mice into two groups: those that were fed CoQ10 and those that were not. The mice that ingested CoQ10 in their diets lived twice as long as those devoid of the nutrient and much longer than mice normally live. Dr. Bliznakov also noted that the mice taking CoQ10 also appeared to have brighter eyes and shinier fur, and lacked the signs of advanced aging.[14] Other studies indicate that CoQ10 is important in increasing energy levels, preventing heart disease, and strengthening the immune system.[15]

So you may be wondering about minerals and their role with regard to enzymes. As you learned earlier, many minerals are required by the body for critical metabolic and life functions. While not specifically considered coenzymes, they are needed to ensure proper enzyme function in your body. As a result, they are sometimes called cofactors. Minerals like magnesium support the proper functioning of hundreds of enzymes in your body—all of which are needed for a vibrant and healthy body. Minerals help to ensure that enzymes can adequately break down protein into amino acids, fats into fatty acids, and carbohydrates into sugar for energy. Let's take a look at just a few minerals and their supportive roles with enzymes.

Zinc is involved in at least 300 enzyme activities in your body, particularly those that metabolize carbohydrates, alcohol, and fatty acids. Zinc also works with the pancreatic enzymes, many of which cannot perform their functions without this important nutrient. As if that weren't enough for this single nutrient, zinc also plays a critical role in the functioning of the powerful antioxidant enzyme, superoxide dismutase (or SOD as it is also known). SOD is one of the body's best defences against aging and disease. Some studies also indicate that SOD shows promise in combatting heart disease.[16]

Magnesium plays a cofactor role in over 500 enzymes in the body, including in those linked to energy metabolism and the synthesis of fats, protein, and genetic material. Many functions of metabolism simply would not occur or would not occur properly without adequate magnesium. Yet some experts estimate that 80 percent of the population may be deficient in this important mineral. That could be a component of our obesity epidemic. What's more, magnesium is essential in many of the coenzyme functions linked to vitamin B1.

Why We Need More Enzyme-Rich Food

Our internal capacity to produce enzymes has greatly diminished even by the age of 35. Some experts estimate that 80 percent of people over the age of 35 are suffering from "enzyme exhaustion." Our pancreas and liver simply cannot keep up with the high demands we place on these overburdened organs. The good news is that by eating more foods in their natural state—or with the enzymes still intact— we can restore digestion and metabolism, and give the pancreas and liver a much-needed break. The result: more energy. And more energy translates into a stronger immune system, improved disease resistance, a speedier metabolism, and possibly even a longer life!

By simply following the life force diet, you'll increase the enzyme-rich foods in your body and reap the countless rewards that life force enzymes offer.

PART TWO

Living With Life Force

4

Week One—Dump the 3 Ps

"I went into a McDonald's yesterday and said,
'I'd like some fries.' The girl at the counter
said, 'Would you like some fries with that?'"

—Jay Leno

THERE are many quotations I could use to start this chapter on the life force diet program but this one stands out for me. It illustrates just how mindless our approach to food can be, whether we are serving it or eating it. Think of the last time you sat down to a quick meal at a local fast food restaurant or opted for the drive-through window as you rushed back to the office. You probably don't remember tasting the food you bought, let alone enjoying it. As my husband said, much to my dismay, when I met him, "I only eat because I have to." That wouldn't be so bad if the food of choice was healthy. Too often our choices are not. We'll be exploring common eating habits and choices in this chapter, which begins the first week of the life force diet.

During this week (or longer if you prefer to take longer to implement the three phases of the life force diet) I'll be asking you to start making important dietary and lifestyle changes. But I never ask people to do something that they don't first understand. When people understand the rationale behind making healthier choices, the choices not only become easier, they also become longer lasting. During this week, you'll discover the foods that are damaging your body and sabotaging your efforts for balanced weight and great health. And, of course, you'll eliminate those foods from your diet.

If your diet consisted primarily of junk foods, you may actually want to eliminate these foods as well as implementing some of the suggestions in the next chapter. That's perfectly fine. Or you can eliminate the junk this week and wait until next week to add the Life Force Silver Foods that are jam-packed with nutrients you'll learn about in the next chapter. Finally, in week three, you'll be making 50 percent of your diet Life Force Gold Foods—Nature's crowning glory of healing and weight-loss wonders.

The life force diet begins as a three-week program because research shows that after 21 days of making a change in our lives, it has become habit. And that's exactly what I'm hoping the life force diet will be for you—a great habit that you continue for the rest of your life. While people lose weight on this program, it is not like other diets in that it is meant to be a new way of life, not a crash diet that you couldn't and wouldn't want to sustain for life. The life force diet will help you achieve a balanced weight, prevent and even reverse many diseases...and who wouldn't want to experience that all life long? But even if you set out to partake for only three weeks, I anticipate that you'll feel so much better that you'll decide to keep going.

Throughout the next few chapters you'll find text boxes called "Ignite Your Life Force" that explain the exact steps you need to take to experience the health benefits of the life force diet. Dive right into the suggestions contained in these boxes to start experiencing more life force right now. These "Ignite Your Life Force" boxes are your at-a-glance guide to following the life force diet without having to wade through volumes of text or make countless notes to remember the program. I still encourage you to read the surrounding text in the next chapters to have a better understanding of the lifestyle and dietary changes you'll be making. You can also flip back through these chapters to re-read the text boxes as a quick reminder of the things you should be doing to follow the life force diet program. I'm sure you're eager to get started, so here's the first "Ignite Your Life Force" step:

Ignite Your Life Force

STEP 1   Drink Up!

If you're not already drinking 8 to 10 cups of pure water daily, now is the time to start. As you learned earlier, your cells, tissues, and organs need water to perform their countless functions. Building life force requires adequate water.

On the road? Take a stainless steel water bottle.

At a desk all day? Just keep a bottle or pitcher of water there too so you'll remember to drink up.

Need more reminders? No problem—set a timer on your computer, watch, or PDA to "go off" every hour to remind you to drink another cup of water.

If you're drinking coffee or tea, now is the time to cut back to one cup of organic coffee or tea a day. And don't forget to add 2 more cups of water to replace fluids lost for each caffeinated beverage.

Give your liver and brain a break by eliminating alcohol for the next few weeks. After that you can enjoy an occasional drink.

Does Your Diet Build a Healthy Body?

You now understand the importance of adequate fresh air and water. And you now know that your body also needs many different nutrients that must be obtained from food, and are dependent on a sound digestive system. In Chapter 2, you learned some of the essential nutrients and nutritional factors that you need to be eating to have a healthy and energetic body. You also learned that most people's diets do not provide adequate quantities of key nutrients and nutritional factors and are actually on the opposite side of the spectrum. That is, most people eat mindlessly or for taste alone, and the incidence of obesity and serious disease is showing it. Let's examine the typical person's diet to determine whether it provides the raw materials needed at the cellular level for your body to perform optimally, or conversely, causes toxic build-up in the cells and tissues.

According to recent information from the U.S. National Center for Health Statistics, 30 percent of Americans are obese—approximately 60 million people. Another third of the population is overweight. Plus the percentage of obese children has tripled in less than 30 years. The Centers for Disease Control and Prevention (CDC) indicate that over 9 million children and teens between the ages of 6 and 19 are overweight.

In Canada, the numbers are only modestly better with 23 percent of adults in the obese category and 26.2 percent of children between age 2 and 17 either overweight or obese. Europeans and Asians are experiencing a growing obesity problem as well. Fortunately, eating for taste does not have to lead to poor nutritional choices and obesity.

Living the life force way requires minimal effort to achieve maximum results. I've designed the life force diet to be a simple step-by-step approach to healthy eating during which time I hope you will be empowered to make lasting changes to your diet. Once you feel the surge of energy and the health that is truly possible for your body, I am confident that you'll always want to feel that great!

The 3 Ps Pack a Nasty Punch

The next step of the life force diet is to eliminate what I call "The 3 Ps"—processed, packaged, and prepared foods. Of course, not all packaged foods need to be avoided. There are many foods that need to be packaged to be shipped and sold, such as oils, vinegars, rice, pasta noodles, and breads. Avoid the ones that contain colours, preservatives, trans- or hydrogenated fats, dairy products, or sweeteners (anything that ends in "–ose"). Certain sweeteners are allowed on the life force diet and they include: stevia rebaudiana (usually just labeled "stevia"), agave nectar, pure maple syrup, or unpasteurized honey. While stevia can be used extensively on the diet, the other sweeteners should be limited to small amounts—a teaspoon at a time, a few times a day, particularly if you're trying to lose weight. Life force condiments include: extra virgin olive oil, coconut oil, cold-pressed grapeseed oil, sesame oil (in small quantities), apple cider vinegar (with the "mother" left in), organic balsamic or wine vinegar, tahini (sesame butter), nut butters, and 100 percent fruit jams. And, don't forget that you can sprinkle raw, unsalted nuts and seeds over any food, so that includes: pine nuts, walnuts, almonds, Brazil nuts, pistachios, hazelnuts, or any other nut you might enjoy as well as sesame, pumpkin, sunflower, hemp, or other types of seeds.

If you're wondering which of these three Ps to avoid, I suggest you visit your local grocery store. I would bet that at least 85 percent of the shelves, freezers, and displays contain processed, packaged, and pre-processed packaged, and prepared foods that contain food additives, refined sugars and salt, unhealthy fats, preservatives, and colourings. Before you panic that you will somehow be sacrificing great taste and all your favourite foods, rest assured that you will soon learn about healthy and tasty alternatives to some of your favourite "P" foods. There are some delicious treasures in the other 15 percent of the store! I'll even share some of my secrets about how to eliminate food cravings for the worst offenders. And by eliminating the 3 Ps, you will be eliminating on average 124 pounds of food additives and reducing 150 pounds of sugar, 8 pounds of salt, and 5 pounds of trans fats from your diet every year! That alone makes this program a must for better health and longevity.

You don't need to worry. Getting the 3 Ps out of your diet is easier than it seems. And you don't have to sacrifice taste. You can still enjoy many of your favourite foods. You can take as little time or as much time as you'd like to implement this first step. Some people do better to jump head first and eliminate all the junk food from their diet, while others need a more gradual approach. Unlike the one-size-fits-all approaches found in other programs, the life force diet is adjustable to suit your particular needs and lifestyle. It is my belief that a flexible approach works best.

Flexibility Is All in Your Mind

Throughout *The Life Force Diet*, it is also imperative to keep an open mind. Let me share a story with you to demonstrate how important an open mind can be.

A book reviewer of my recent book, *The Ultimate pH Solution*, gave the book quite a positive review; then she went on to comment on the use of avocado in my pudding recipes. I'm a big fan of making pudding using the protein-packed, essential fatty acid-endowed and nutrient-rich avocado since it lends a creamy texture while being a superb Life Force Gold Food. She felt that she could never "trick" herself into thinking that pudding made with avocado was really pudding. Like most people, she believed that there is only one "right" way to prepare certain foods.

We've become so accustomed to one way of doing things or one way of eating that we think it is the only way. Many of the recipes are healthier versions of some of your favourites. They are made following healthier food preparation principles. Changing the way they're made does not affect their wonderful taste. Actually, many people have written to me to tell me they just love the taste of my pudding recipes. I've even had world-renowned physicians like Dr. Michael Roizen, author of the best-selling book *You: The Owner's Manual* and the similarly named radio show, sing the praises of my recipes! Give them a try ... you might be surprised.

Real Food Doesn't Come with Labels

When was the last time you read the label on something you bought? Or requested the ingredient information on your fast-food favourites? If you did, you were probably more than a bit uncomfortable with the names of scary-sounding ingredients. And you should be. As you learned earlier, we're eating about 124 pounds of hidden chemical additives in our food every year—none of which should be eaten as part of a healthy diet.

Real food doesn't contain harmful monosodium glutamate, sodium benzoate, FD & C number 5, or any number of other concoctions whipped up in a laboratory. I tell all my clients that if you can't pronounce it or recognize it, it probably isn't food and your body probably doesn't need it. Real food has no need for labels. Instead of these nasty ingredients, Mother Nature's finest fruits, vegetables, nuts, seeds, and grains will make up the bulk of your diet.

You probably still have questions about what constitutes "real food." As you read through the book, you are going to learn all about real food, how to prepare it, and what it does to make you feel great. Right now, I'm going to tell you what real food is *not,* so you'll better understand some of the foods you need to avoid or at least reconsider as dietary choices. Let's start with some of our misconceptions about protein and meat, as well as calcium and dairy. I'll also tell you why sugar and sugar substitutes are as harmful as many drugs and why you need to learn about good carbohydrates and good fats (we eat too many bad carbs and bad fats). Finally, I will guide you through the dangers of additives, colours, pesticides, and genetically modified foods.

Ignite Your Life Force

> **STEP 2** **Read That Label!**
> While some nutrients have long-winded scientific names, the vast majority of hard-to-pronounce ingredients are things you really shouldn't be eating—things that are dragging your life force down.

So grab a garbage bag, open your fridge and start tossing anything with ingredients you can't pronounce, haven't heard of, or that you know shouldn't be in your body. And, if you're not sure, throw it out. This is the time to get totally honest with yourself—anything containing F D & C yellow number 5 has no place in your fridge, let alone in your body. And just because you recognize sodium as salt doesn't mean you should keep something containing sodium benzoate. For future grocery orders, read labels. Better yet, buy real food that doesn't need a label—you'll find it in the produce section of your grocery store.

Protein—Beyond the Meat Myth

Most foods contain protein, including fruits and vegetables, yet many people still believe the myth that meat is the best or only source of protein. This myth and the dietary habits that support it are having serious health ramifications.

The average North American eats over 248 pounds of meat every year. That's about 40 percent of his or her diet. Most experts confirm that meat should not exceed about 10 percent of our overall food intake. So the average person is eating four times the amount he or she needs. Our ancestors ate only about 5 percent of their total food intake in the form of meat. And they ate substantially less food than we're eating.

While the proponents of high-protein diets espouse their weight-loss capacity, the reality is that almost everyone is currently on a high-protein diet just because of excessive meat consumption. And the overweight and obesity statistics, as you read earlier, are staggering.

The potential health risks of obesity are much greater than simply being overweight. According to the CDC, being overweight or obese is a factor in many health conditions, including high cholesterol or high triglycerides; endometrial, breast, and colon cancers; gallbladder disease; heart disease; hypertension; osteoarthritis; sleep apnea and respiratory problems; stroke; and type 2 diabetes. And one of the things proponents of high protein diets won't tell you is that excess protein in your diet is turned into glucose (sugar) or glycogen (a specific type of sugar that is made in the liver and muscles in your body), or turned into fat. That's right: too much protein is stored as fat!

In Denmark back in 1917, the government stopped feeding the nation's supply of grain to livestock that would be later killed and used for meat. Instead, they fed the grain directly to Danish people. Something surprising happened: When the mortality rate was calculated for that year, they discovered that the overall death rate from disease was the lowest in their recorded history.[1] The researchers attributed the change to the reduced meat intake.

Now I'm not suggesting our governments reallocate livestock feed for human consumption, but you get the point. We're simply eating way too much meat.

But it's not just the quantity of protein foods that play a role in health—the quality of the protein is also important. Animal protein requires a massive amount of energy and plentiful amounts of digestive juices and enzymes to adequately break down the meat into its amino acid constituent components. The result: Excessive meat can be hard on the digestive system and your whole body. And depending on the strength of your digestive system, even a small amount of concentrated protein foods like meat may be difficult for your body to break down, meaning your body may not be getting the important amino acids contained within the protein food. Everyone is unique in this regard. Meat is also devoid of fibre and contains little water, both of which are needed to ensure the proper movement of foods through the digestive tract. Excess meat can slow the whole process and potentially lead to waste and toxins being absorbed through the walls of your intestines alongside the nutrients that normally follow this path. Additionally, the by-products of meat digestion are acidic and can put a strain on the kidneys to eliminate the acid.

I'm not suggesting that everyone eliminate all forms of meat, poultry, and fish from their diet, although many people would do well to do so. Certainly it is possible to be extremely healthy on a vegetarian diet, but many people find it difficult to maintain for extended periods. I encourage people to go vegetarian or to become as close to vegetarian as they are comfortable with while on the life force diet. The reality is that some people feel better when they eat a small amount of meat, while others thrive on vegetarianism.

Regardless, if you're eating a typical North American diet, you're eating far too much meat. And, if your meat consists of burgers from your local fast-food joint, you're not getting the best quality of meat. Most of our meat supply is now contaminated with antibiotics, hormones, and preservatives never intended for human consumption. And all of these less-than-desirables can disrupt the body's delicate hormonal and nervous systems.

So, eat no more than about 15 percent of your daily diet as lean meat, poultry, fish, or eggs. While many people may believe that they need more than that, there is no evidence to suggest that is true. I encourage the consumption of low-toxin, high-nutrient fish such as wild salmon since it provides some important fatty acids that can be difficult to get on an exclusively vegetarian diet. But choose only low-toxin fish (like wild salmon) since farmed varieties typically have high amounts of the banned pesticides PCBs, DDT, and the hazardous heavy metal, mercury. Also, choose only organic meat, poultry, and eggs to avoid the dangerous antibiotics and hormones used in conventional practices.

Ignite Your Life Force

> ### STEP 3   Limit Your Meat Consumption
> Limit your intake of all types of animal protein to no more than 15 percent of your diet. Yes, that includes white meat, red meat, and any other type of meat, including fish, and eggs. That means

taking a look at your plate and making sure that only about one-seventh of the food you're eating is meat. And try to choose only organic meat free of antibiotics, hormones, or other unwanted ingredients. Remember: You are what you eat! And, don't worry if you don't like meat or prefer to go vegetarian. That's a valid option on the life force diet.

When Dairy Goes Bad

In the same way we've become accustomed to thinking of meat as the only food source of protein, we've come to think of dairy products as the only source of calcium. This myth is having detrimental effects on our health. Dairy products are not health foods, contrary to what dairy boards and their milk-moustache-wearing celebrities may suggest. There's no question that milk and other dairy products contain calcium. But just because milk contains calcium does not mean that your body will absorb the calcium, nor does it mean that it is a healthy food option. Laboratory conditions used to determine the amount of calcium in dairy products are simply not the same as the conditions inside the human body.

Other than domestic animals to which we feed cow's milk, humans are the only species that consumes the milk of another species. And that's long after we're supposedly weaned from milk consumption as infants. Cow's milk is simply not suitable for human consumption. A cow has four chambers in its stomach to help it to digest its mother's milk. A human being has only two stomach chambers, which is insufficient to adequately break down the milk protein.

Our modern cow's milk supply is laden with growth hormones used to fatten cattle and lengthen the duration of lactation, antibiotics used to ward off animal infections, and residue of other medications that they may have consumed.

The United States and Canada have two of the highest rates of osteoporosis in the world, yet North Americans drink more milk and eat more cheese and ice cream than most other countries in the world.

If you need more convincing, consider the environmental implications of raising meat and dairy cattle. As more parts of the world, including the American Mid-West, experience extended droughts, water is becoming an increasingly precious resource. The amount of water required to raise beef and dairy cattle is staggering, especially in contrast to the amount required to grow an equivalent measure of vegetables.

It's important to wean yourself off dairy products this week of the life force diet and continue to avoid them throughout the program. For most people, the more they avoid dairy products, the better they typically feel. This is especially true for anyone with allergies, breathing disorders, and pain disorders like arthritis, since many people have hidden food sensitivities to dairy products that are creating the symptoms of these illnesses.

There are many good milk substitutes, such as almond milk, rice milk, and in some cases soy milk (read about the pros and cons of soy in the next chapter). They don't taste the same as cow's milk, but have their own delicious tastes. If you don't like one particular variety, try another one, since the taste varies between varieties and brands.

Ignite Your Life Force

> **STEP 4   Dump the Dairy**
>
> Milk is for calves, not humans. It's time to ditch the dairy products. Yes, that means all dairy products: milk, cheese, cottage cheese, yogurt, sour cream, ice cream, and even "cheese substitutes" that contain casein or other dairy ingredients. Your life force will thank you! Use almond milk or rice milk in your baking, on your cereal, or to make smoothies. Don't expect them to taste the same as cow's milk—they have their own delicious taste.

Sugar Overload: Depressed and Suppressed

I was in my favourite café recently, enjoying a tea and doing research for this book when a family entered the building. It appeared that the parents and their two young children had spent the early afternoon outdoors at the tulip festival and were in need of a snack. The kids quietly waited while the parents ordered lattes for themselves and bottled juices and cookies for the kids. I returned to my reading only to be interrupted within 10 minutes by screaming children, running around the café. The parents, halfway through their lattes, clearly had no energy left to maintain order. I waited, knowing what would happen next. Another 10 minutes passed and the kids quieted down ... somewhat. They started to whine and complain to their parents. They became sullen and the younger one started to cry. They were victims of a sugar high and low.

On average, we eat well over 2½ pounds of sugar weekly, adding up to over 150 pounds of sugar annually in the form of sugary soft drinks, so-called juices, cookies, cakes, and pastries, and hidden in processed and prepared foods. Compare that to our ancestors just over 100 years ago: They ate only 5 pounds of sugar annually.

Linked to high blood pressure, high cholesterol, heart disease, weight gain, diabetes, and premature aging, to name only a few, sugar in the amounts we consume is one of the worst substances we put into our bodies. Even a fairly small amount suppresses your immune system for between four and six hours, giving any viruses or bacteria you've been exposed to a heady advantage to take hold of your body.

If you're suffering from hormonal imbalances, depression, or allergies look no further than to that chocolate cake, cola, and ice cream you recently consumed, since sugar is linked to all of these health concerns. Sugar has even been linked to cancer.

From ketchup and burgers to salt and juice, sugar may be lurking in the most unlikely places. But the worst culprit is soft drinks. According to the Center for Science in the Public Interest, enough money is spent on soft drinks in America to supply every man, woman, and child in America with 587 servings of the sugary stuff every year. And each can of soft drinks contains between 7 and 11 teaspoons of sugar.

Teenagers are consuming almost 10 percent of their total food and beverage caloric intake as soft drinks. This is a habit that's gotten way out of hand. And research shows that the white powder is more addictive than cocaine, which could explain our out-of-control habit and our need to start breaking it.[2]

Here's the good news: Sugar consumption is easy to reduce because we are starting from such a high quantity. This week and throughout the life force diet, eliminate soft drinks. If you are thirsty, drink water, herbal tea, or vegetable juice (be careful of the bottled brands—they can be full of sugar and salt too). If you have a sweet tooth, reach for a piece of fruit. I find a delicious blend of green tea lemonade made with freshly squeezed lemon and sweetened only with stevia to be a great thirst quencher. But remember, replacing sugar with most sugar substitutes is replacing one poison with another.

Ignite Your Life Force

STEP 5 · Kick the Sugar Habit

Consuming excess sugar in its myriad forms is a sure-fire way to watch your life force plummet. If you haven't already thrown out anything in your cupboards or fridge that contains sweeteners of any kind, now is the time to do so. If you're not sure, look for any ingredient that contains "-ose" such as glucose, high fructose corn syrup, dextrose, maltose, etc. Instead, use small amounts (maximum 1 teaspoon three times a day) of pure, unpasteurized honey, pure maple syrup, barley malt, agave nectar, or the herb stevia. Stevia is the best choice and the only one that doesn't affect blood sugar levels. It is between 300 and 1000 times sweeter than sugar, depending on whether you're using the whole herb or the liquid extract. I use a liquid extract since I find it has the best taste and less aftertaste. You can use it in fresh juices like lemon or lime juice with water to make a delicious lemonade or limeade, or to sweeten herbal teas—either hot or iced ones instead of soft drinks—and even in baking (although most recipes will need ingredient adjustments when using stevia).

The Sugar-Free Fallacy

So, you may be thinking, "I avoid sugar by choosing healthier sugar-free foods and beverages." Well, you may be shocked to learn the truth about the artificial sweeteners behind the "sugar-free" labels: They're not the healthy stuff their manufacturers claim them to be. Actually, they're even worse.

The chemical sweeteners include saccharin, aspartame, and, more recently, sucralose. You may know them better as Sweet 'N Low, Sugar Twin, NutraSweet, Equal, Sunnett, Sweet One, and Splenda. Sugar substitutes may go by many names and taste as sweet as their sugary counterpart, but they are linked to an even longer list of health disorders.

Let's explore aspartame first. It is made primarily of aspartic acid, phenylalanine, and methanol. Our bodies lack the enzymes to break down toxic methanol. Instead, our bodies convert it into the carcinogen formaldehyde. Scientific studies link aspartame consumption to a lengthy list of health problems, which include anxiety, brain tumours, birth defects, depression, epilepsy, learning disabilities, menstrual irregularities, migraines, psychiatric disorders, premenstrual syndrome, psychiatric disorders, and reproductive problems.[3]

Only 15 studies examined the safety of the sugar substitute sucralose, or Splenda, as it is primarily known (incidentally, 13 of these 15 studies were funded by the manufacturer itself). In seven of these studies sucralose was linked to migraines.[4] The largest study involved only 138 people over 13 weeks. So we really don't know the long-term effects of sucralose consumption—unless you consider 13 weeks long term. That is definitely inadequate for its rampant and lengthy use in North America.

Sugar substitutes offer no value in your diet, and worse than that, are likely impeding your ability to experience vibrant health. They need to be eliminated on the life force diet.

Ignite Your Life Force

> **STEP 6** Sugar Substitutes? Just Say No!
>
> If you're eating sugar substitutes, even ones supposedly "made from real sugar," now is the time to kick the aspartame, lose the sucralose, and shun every food containing artificial sweeteners. No exceptions.

Bad Carbs, Good Carbs

So how can you possibly satisfy a sweet tooth or provide energy for your body without eating excessive amounts of sugar or artificial sweeteners? Your body needs some carbs. It just needs the right kind. Complex carbohydrates, also known as "healthy carbohydrates," are found in whole grains and foods made from them, as well as vegetables and fruit. These healthy carbs digest slower than refined sugars thanks to the fibre naturally found in them. Once digested, the natural sugars found in these carbs provide the main source of energy in our bodies. The fibre content ensures a slow and steady release of these sugars as fuel, while preventing blood sugar spikes and drops that cause energy crashes, mood swings, irritability, jitteriness, or other symptoms of low blood sugar, also known as "hypoglycemia." Many people have been informed by their doctors that they are hypoglycemic. I remind people that if you tested a healthy person's blood sugar if they haven't eaten anything for several hours (like most of us do when we get busy) or after they've eaten refined sugars or its many forms like pastries, sugary cereals, cola, or other common foods in our diet, that person would show up as being hypoglycemic. Remember, "hypoglycemic" means "under-sweet-blood" or "low blood sugar." While it can be a serious condition, more often it reflects poor food choices or eating habits.

Without healthy carbs our cells wouldn't have the energy they need to function at all. We'll be discussing some excellent complex carbohydrates that you'll want to include in your diet in the coming chapters, and feel free to flip ahead and start including some of these healthy carb options this week if you want to.

Ignite Your Life Force

> **STEP 7** **Kick the Refined Carbs**
>
> There's no place for white bread, refined cereals, and white pasta on the life force diet, especially when spelt bread, oatmeal, and brown rice pasta are so readily available and taste better too. Eliminate all foods made with white flour or its other guises: wheat flour, semolina flour (or just semolina), durum wheat flour, or 100 percent wheat flour. These carbs are refined and are treated similarly to white sugar in the body. Choose bread, cereal, or pasta made from Life Force Silver Foods like oats, spelt, kamut, millet, brown rice, wild rice, or quinoa, which we'll discuss in greater detail in the next chapter.

Clogging Your Body with Damaging Fats

Your body needs essential fatty acids from foods that contain fat to use as energy, to insulate the body and protect the organs, including the brain, from damage. There are numerous types of fats and, unfortunately, most people are choosing foods that contain harmful fats and not enough of the foods that contain beneficial fatty acids. Most of the fat found in the typical diet comes from fried foods, cooking oils, margarine, shortening, lard, meat, and foods or processed foods made from these ingredients. Trans fats are the worst type of fat people are ingesting. Currently, the average person eats 5 pounds of trans fats per year.[5] Any amount of trans fats in your diet can potentially cause health concerns.

Most of the trans fats we consume are artificially manufactured by industry to lengthen the shelf life (and increase profits) of fats and foods containing them. They are manufactured by adding hydrogen atoms to unsaturated fats to make them more saturated. Saturated simply refers to whether a fat molecule is full of hydrogen atoms or not. Most naturally occurring saturated fats are found in meats and animal fat like lard and are linked to heart disease and other health concerns. One of the exceptions is coconut oil, which contains high levels of saturated fats but is actually health-promoting. I'll explain more about why coconut oil is the exception and the health benefits linked to it in the coming chapters.

Ignite Your Life Force

> **STEP 8** **Eliminate the 3 Ps**
>
> If you haven't already eliminated the 3 Ps, processed, prepared, and packaged food, now is the time to do so. By eliminating these "foods" you'll avoid most trans fats, hidden sugar, preservatives, colours, and other additives that destroy your life force.

Healthy fats that contain beneficial fatty acids are essential for the production and movement of energy throughout the body. They even help to transport the oxygen you inhale to the cells and are imperative to healthy blood clotting if you cut or injure your body. These essential fatty acids, or EFAs as they are also known, support a healthy immune system so you can fend off viruses and other micro-organisms. A particular type of essential fatty acids called Omega 3s play a critical role in reducing inflammation that is linked to aging, and protecting the nervous system and brain. A deficiency can impair learning and mental capacity and is linked to depression, attention deficit disorder, and autism.

The trans fats I mention above are particularly damaging to the brain. They actually take the place of healthy fats in cellular membranes in both the brain and nerve cells when we don't eat enough of the healthy fats listed below. Not only do trans fats impair the brain directly, researchers speculate that their composition makes them less capable of blocking toxins from crossing the blood-brain barrier, a critical defence mechanism designed to allow nutrients to enter the brain while blocking many harmful substances and pathogens. Conversely, healthy fats make the brain less permeable to toxins like heavy metals and viruses.

To complicate matters, the trans fats are substituted at a one-to-one ratio in place of healthy fats, according to researchers. Worse than that, in the absence of healthy Omega 3 fatty acids, you can absorb up to twice as many trans fats. Simply put, you aren't getting any Omega 3s when you eat the 3Ps—donuts, cookies, French fries, and most snack foods. But you are getting a heck of a lot of trans fats. The same is true with most cooking oils, including those billed as "healthy" alternatives—canola, sunflower, safflower, and vegetable oils.

Speaking of ratios, the typical person's diet, if it contains any healthy essential fatty acids, usually includes fat found in meat and poultry, or healthier fats from nuts and seeds called Omega 6 fatty acids. Both Omega 3s and Omega 6s are critical to great health, but need to be found in our diets in a healthy ratio such as one-to-one or two-to-one in favour of Omega 6s. However, the average person eats these foods in a 20-to-1 to a 40-to-1 ratio, causing a significant excess of Omega 6s and insufficient Omega 3s, thereby resulting in insufficient Omega 3s to keep inflammation in our bodies in check. Wild salmon, flaxseeds and flax oil, and raw walnuts are all great sources of Omega 3s. Increasing these foods, while decreasing foods made with canola oil (which is typically genetically modified and excessively heated during processing), for example, will help you restore a healthy ratio.

Because you're eliminating the 3 Ps, you'll eliminate most, if not all, trans fats from your diet. By reducing your meat consumption or foregoing it altogether, you'll dramatically reduce your intake of saturated fats. Start cooking with pure coconut oil and extra virgin olive oil (alternating them) to increase your intake in healthy fats. Avoid deep-fried foods. Sauté your food on low to medium heat instead. Or choose baking or steaming as healthy cooking options.

Ignite Your Life Force

> **STEP 9** **When Smoke Gets in Your Eyes**
>
> Make sure your cooking oil and any food cooked in oil never smokes (steam is okay and you'll know the difference by the smell as well as the appearance). Even healthy oil becomes unhealthy when it reaches the "smoke point." If it smokes, throw it out.

A Grain of Salt

We're also eating excessive amounts of salt. While your body needs sodium to ensure the proper regulation of blood and bodily fluids, to transmit electrical impulses within the brain and between the brain and nervous system, to control heart activity, and for certain metabolic functions, we're getting far too much in our diet. The average person eats about 10 grams of sodium daily but needs only about 3 grams. That adds up to about 8 pounds of salt per year. The lion's share (about 75 percent) of the sodium we ingest is found in the 3 Ps: the processed, packaged, or prepared foods we are eating. Experts suggest that cutting our sodium intake by 2 grams would save about 10,000 lives from heart attacks and strokes every year.[6]

Excess sodium allows too much water to enter into our cells, creating a higher pressure inside. Essentially, that heavy, bloated feeling many of us feel goes all the way down to the cellular level inside our bodies and is at least in part due to excess sodium intake. By eliminating the 3 Ps from your diet, you'll likely be reducing your sodium intake to within healthy limits. That is, unless you go overboard with the salt shaker. Throw out the iodized or table salt and instead fill your salt shaker with Himalayan crystal salt (a slightly orangey colour) or Celtic sea salt (slightly greyish colour). Both of these better salt options are readily available in your health food store. Still, go easy on your salt intake.

Ignite Your Life Force

> **STEP 10** The Salt of the Earth
>
> Switch to Celtic sea salt or Himalayan crystal salt instead of the standard table salt and you'll immediately reduce your sodium intake. Both of these healthier options contain less sodium and higher amounts of other minerals, including potassium, making them a healthier option. Can't find either? Look for a greyish, moist-looking salt at your local health food store instead.
>
> Celery seeds (not celery salt, which is just celery-flavoured salt) make a great alternative to salt when cooking soups, stews, chili, or other foods. It has a naturally salty flavour but is great for reducing pain and inflammation in your body thanks to its 20 anti-pain and anti-inflammatory compounds! I keep a bottle of celery seeds in a salt shaker ready for immediate use while cooking.

Fast Food, Fake Food

I know I said it earlier but it is worth repeating: The average person eats over 124 pounds of chemical food additives every year.[7] The food manufacturing industry adds them to food for many purposes, making it common to find multiple types of food additives in any processed, packaged, or prepared foods. Some of the more than 3000 additives used[8] include acid/base balancers, bleach, colours, conditioners, firming agents, flavours, flavour enhancers, heavy metals, nutrient enrichers, preservatives, ripening gases, and texture agents.[9] These chemicals add no value, no nutrients, and no health benefits. Conversely, many of these chemicals are known neurotoxins, meaning that they are damaging to your brain and nervous system. Some are a specific class of neurotoxins called excitotoxins that literally excite your brain cells to death. With the high consumption of these excitotoxins, is there any wonder that there is an alarming increase of children suffering from developmental disorders such as attention deficit hyperactivity disorder (ADHD) and autism? I believe these types of disorders are closely linked to the increase in harmful chemicals in our food.

The body of research on some of these additives, such as colourings, continues to grow and, with the exception of studies funded by the food processing industry, illustrate the health dangers and other potential dangers of these chemicals. Other chemicals, such as "food flavours," have not been sufficiently assessed and are still flying under the radar for the most part. If you have to synthetically add flavour to something to pass it off as food, maybe it shouldn't be classified as food in the first place.

Ignite Your Life Force

STEP 11 Can the Soda

By now, you should have already eliminated soda from your diet. High in sugars or artificial sweeteners, colours, and preservatives, this beverage is a serious destroyer of your life force. If you haven't cut out the cola or other carbonated beverages, do so now. Your body will reward you in the form of greater energy, vitality, and greater protection against disease. Opt for Life Force Lemonade (see the recipes at the back of this book), iced herbal teas, fresh juices, or pure water.

MSG, Good Enzymes, and Bad Enzymes

Monosodium glutamate (MSG) is the most commonly known excitotoxin. MSG, short for mono-sodium glutamate, is made up of sodium and an amino acid that are chemically altered to create a substance that the body cannot adequately deal with.

MSG consumption is linked to obesity, asthma attacks, headaches, heart irregularities, hives, insomnia, panic attacks, seizures, and many other symptoms.[10] It may also be linked to Alzheimer's and Parkinson's disease.[11]

A study conducted by scientists at the Department of Biochemistry in Panjab University and reported in the *Indian Journal of Clinical Biochemistry* found that ingestion of MSG at a dose level of 4 milligrams or more per gram of weight in mice resulted in oxidative stress due to an increase in a free radical initiating substance called xanthine oxidase. Not only did the MSG significantly increase this unhealthy substance, it significantly decreased the activity of beneficial free-radical scavenging enzymes like catalase and superoxide dismutase in the liver tissue—two important enzymes needed to protect the body from damage.[12] Other studies on mice link MSG to damaged nerve cells.[13]

Because MSG is used as a "flavour enhancer" in soups, bottled salad dressings, chips, and other processed, packaged, and prepared foods, you'll be substantially lessening your potential exposure by eliminating the 3 Ps from your diet, which you begin this week and continue throughout the life force diet.

The Dark Side of Colours

The next time you're at a child's birthday party, notice the beautiful array of cakes, cookies, and cupcakes, all showcasing a rainbow assortment of artificial colours. While they may make these sweets look appetizing to children, these synthetic ingredients often take the place of nutrition in foods. For example, fruit juice that contains colours is typically devoid of fruit, making it artificially coloured sugar-water. Worse than that, many food colours are linked to hyperactivity disorders and cancer.[14]

Artificial colouring is a serious problem in fast food and fake food. A recent petition by the Center for Science in the Public Interest, a consumer advocacy group, has called for a ban on the use of artificial dyes in food. The group has targeted its petition at the U.S. Food and Drug Administration, seeking the phasing out of eight artificial food dyes linked to serious health risks. While they have made their case based on the risks to children, I have no doubt these artificial colours are wreaking havoc on adults as well.

While the names of the dyes are meaningless to most people (yellow 5 or tartrazine, which is derived from coal tar, and blue 2 or indigotine, for example), their effects are not. These toxins are commonly found in concentrated fruit juices, condiments, and some cheeses. An article in the *Globe and Mail* reported that many popular snacks such as Smarties, Froot Loops, Cheetos, Doritos and Reeses' Pieces simply list "colours" without defining whether they are from a natural or artificial source.[15]

Blue dye number 1 and 2 are linked with cancer in animal tests, while red dye number 3 causes thyroid tumours in rats. Green dye number 3 is linked to bladder cancer, and yellow dye number 6 is linked to tumours of the kidneys and adrenal glands.[16] While these colours are readily used in most processed, packaged, and prepared foods, what bothers me the most is that they are commonplace in the diets of children. Most candy, cakes, baked goods, maraschino cherries, fruit cocktail, gelatin desserts, and soft drinks contain these harmful substances, which serve no other purpose than to make so-called food look "pretty" and attract children whose bodies are particularly sensitive to them because they are still developing.

While those in the natural health and holistic nutrition fields are aware of the dangers of these dyes, it appears a 2007 study in *The Lancet*, a reputable, mainstream medical journal, brought wider attention to this health concern. Health Canada, the federal government health department, has stated that it has begun to require labelling of colours in food using the specific name, but that doesn't get the toxins out of the food. Knowing what it is doesn't make it less dangerous, only avoidable for those who both read the label and know what to look out for. How many shoppers do that? The food industry must be held accountable for the ingredients they use and strong disincentives are needed to keep dangerous additives and artificial colours out of the food supply.

Preservation at All Costs

The food industry also uses many preservatives in processed, prepared, and packaged foods to maximize shelf life and therefore industry profits. But due to the health effects of these harmful chemicals, they need to be avoided. Sodium nitrate, which is also called sodium nitrite, is a preservative that is added to bacon, ham, luncheon meats, smoked fish, corned beef, and hot dogs. Numerous studies link its consumption to various types of cancer. BHA and BHT, two commonly used preservatives that are short form for butylated hydroxyanisole and butylated hydroxytoluene, are found in breakfast cereals, chewing gum, vegetable oils, and potato chips. They can cause oxidative damage in the body, which is a nice way of saying "premature aging." Research shows that they form potentially cancer-causing substances in the body.[17] Propyl gallate is another preservative that is typically used alongside BHA and BHT in soup bases, meat products, and chewing gum. It may also be carcinogenic.[18] Potassium bromate sounds like it might be a healthy mineral, but it's actually a harmful additive that is used in bread, buns, and other baked goods but is known to cause cancer in animals and increase the risk of cancer in humans.[19]

By eliminating the 3 Ps you'll substantially reduce or eliminate MSG and other toxic flavour enhancers, health-damaging food colours, and cancer-causing preservatives.

Stay Away from the Spray

Over time as research unfolds, humankind may look back with regret on the decision to spray our food with pesticides.

Did you know that a common class of pesticides called organo-phosphates originated as nerve agents developed during World War I? When there was no longer a need for them in warfare, industry adapted them to kill pests on food. So it should come as no surprise that some of these chemicals are toxic to our nervous system and brains. Some are also carcinogenic.

I am always astounded when I walk by a medical office or a health centre and I see the signs on the lawn that state, "Warning: Pesticide Use." It is bad enough that the general public continues to use these chemicals, let alone professionals who should really know better. I applaud every community that has taken steps to ban the use of pesticides on public spaces and municipal grounds. A standing ovation to those communities that are banning pesticides altogether!

While you may not be able to avoid pesticides in your community, you can certainly avoid them in your food by choosing organic wherever possible. Not only are organic foods devoid of harmful pesticides, but they are also free of potentially harmful genetically modified ingredients, both of which are excellent reasons to choose organic foods as much as possible. You'll also learn more reasons to choose organic in Chapter 6.

Frankenfoods and Other Freaks of Un-Nature

If the thought of unleashing bacteria shells filled with viruses that spread pesticides in your foods sounds like something out of a scary science fiction movie, think again. This is the stuff of reality. Would you knowingly eat a potato that needs to be transported in hazardous waste containers since every cell contains pesticides? This isn't food terrorism (at least not the kind we recognize as a crime); this is what passes as improvements to our food supply. One day we will learn that we can't improve on nature.

From Flavr Savr tomatoes to Roundup Ready Soybeans, genetically modified foods are being manufactured and unleashed on an unsuspecting public whether we are ready for them or not. The Grocery Manufacturers of America estimates that 75 percent of all processed foods in America contain a genetically modified ingredient.

Governments worldwide should have insisted on extensive safety testing of genetically modified ingredients before allowing them to be unleashed on an unsuspecting public. But the U.S. FDA even states, "The FDA has not found it necessary to conduct comprehensive scientific reviews of foods derived from bioengineered plants ... consistent with its 1992 policy."[20]

Genetically modified (GM) foods are big business in North America, particularly in the United States. They are also supported in Brazil and to a certain extent in Asia. Europe has been appropriately cautious in its approach to GM foods and to date has limited access to the European market, much to the frustration of U.S. business. There is a very real threat that this could change in the near future and the threat is linked to attempted environmentalism.

Recent media reporting has raised the issue of food shortages as crops are diverted to bio-fuel production. In theory, replacing fossil fuels with plant-based alternatives seems like a great idea, and eventually, technology may provide solutions that do not affect the food supply, cause widespread damage to land cleared for "fuel crops," or wipe out indigenous species for the sake of high-yield bio-fuel species.

Supporters of GM foods are exploiting this "crisis" by insisting genetically engineered crops are the only way to deal with the food shortage, to ensure crops can grow on tired, nutrient-weak, drought-susceptible soil (all signs of over-farming and potentially climate-change factors). Lobbyists have seen a crack in Europe's closed door and they have stuck their foot in. Let us hope that the European nations stick to their guns —GM foods have become a global, uncontrolled experiment. The long-term impact is unknown and companies like Monsanto are happy to keep the public and farmers in the dark, playing on their fears of food scarcity, poor harvests, or employing more ominous tactics.

More Problems with Frankenfoods

Did you know 18 percent of all genetically modified seeds have been engineered to produce their own pesticides? That alone makes foods grown from these seeds potentially harmful, but there's more: Research shows that these seeds may continue producing pesticides *inside your body* once you've eaten the food grown from them![21] Those potatoes are sounding even less appetizing now, aren't they?

The food that most people subsist on marginally resembles food as nature intended us to eat. While many of these so-called foods are common in our diets, that does not mean they are normal or healthy or even intended for the human body. These plastic foods, as I refer to the processed, packaged, prepared, refined, irradiated, chemically altered, and genetically modified stuff that comprises the vast majority of what we eat, only act to intoxicate our cells, clog our natural bodily processes, and throw off the balance of our hormones, metabolic functions, detoxification processes, and other body functions.

Here is an example of how this plays out in the body. In today's "youth and beauty" society, aging is practically a crime. But the things

I have discussed in this chapter—the 3Ps, chemicals, additives, and other toxins in our food supply— force our body to work hard processing the junk out of our systems. This processing creates by-products called free radicals in the body. Interestingly, free radicals are also found in pollutants like cigarette smoke and car exhaust. In the body, free radicals damage DNA as well as our tissues, organs, and brain.

The visible result of excessive DNA damage is what we refer to as aging: wrinkles and sagging skin, for example. What we don't see is the damage free radicals do to our internal organs at the cellular level. Each cell is "attacked" by free radicals thousands of times a day and must defend itself. Research shows that after our mid- to late 20s, our capacity to repair DNA damage from free radicals decreases. We start to age more quickly. We aren't helping our cause by ingesting even more free radical–causing substances.

With this basic understanding of how our bodies work, it's easy to understand how our "modern" diet can overstimulate or depress our bodies, mind, and emotions. It is easy to understand how our food and lifestyle choices age us prematurely.

I know you are probably thinking, "This is depressing. What can I eat?" Don't fear; this is actually a good news story. You now know what things are robbing you of your life force. You know what things could be making you tired, sore, overweight, or ill. While the situation sounds bleak, it simply means that making some essential change is likely to result in transformative improvement in your body. And that's where the life force diet can help. This plan will help you to get back in touch with the powerful curative properties of nature and your body's miraculous healing ability.

Your lack of energy, depression, or poor health is not the result of a deficiency in aspirin, of synthetic hormones, or chemotherapy drugs. These substances are merely Band-Aid attempts to eliminate symptoms, but do not address the cause of illness. Our soaring disease rates are the symptom that we are not providing our bodies with the right tools to properly perform the trillions of functions that our bodies are fully capable of handling.

The good news continues in the next chapter. I'm going to introduce you to great foods that will boost your life force, your energy, and your health. As you continue reading, you will discover how easy it is to eat a variety of great-tasting foods—and by foods I'm not talking about packaged, frozen, microwavable, virtually unrecognizable "things" that crowd our grocery aisles and kitchen cupboards.

This is a lifestyle change, not an overnight fix. If you try to go cold turkey, the chances of failure are high. You'll feel like you failed and your motivation will drop. Take it slow, take it steady, and take it seriously. Replace the chocolate bars with fresh fruit. Replace the cola at dinner with water and lemon. Better still, have the water and lemon 40 minutes before you eat and drink less than 4 ounces of liquid with your meal. This will help you digest your food better. Have a meat-free meal at every lunch. When you learn enough recipes in the book, start trying meat-free dinners as well.

Don't worry about treating yourself once in a while. It's not cheating; it's just being human. But you'll probably be surprised and amazed to learn that after a few weeks, those "treats" don't taste quite as good. In fact, you may find them unappetizing. Your palate and your body will change and you will love the results.

Summary: Week 1 of the Life Force Diet

1. Drink up! Drink at least 8 to 10 cups of pure water daily. For every cup of coffee, tea, or alcohol you drink be sure to add an additional 2 cups. Cut alcohol for these first three weeks, and limit yourself to 1 cup of organic coffee or tea per day.

2. Read that label. Eliminate anything that contains suspect ingredients from your diet and household.

3. Limit meat (red meat, poultry, fish, and egg) consumption to a maximum of 15 percent of your total daily diet. Or choose

total vegetarianism. Choose only organic meat, poultry, fish, and eggs, if you're continuing to eat these foods.

4. Dump the dairy. You'll learn some healthy milk substitutes in the next chapter.

5. Kick the sugar habit. And don't forget to eliminate the hidden sugars.

6. Say no to sugar substitutes. Choose only natural sweeteners such as unpasteurized honey, pure maple syrup, agave nectar, barley malt, or rice syrup, or the naturally sweet herb stevia.

7. Kick the refined carbs like white flour and white flour products.

8. Eliminate the 3Ps: packaged, processed, and prepared foods. By doing so, you'll quickly reduce your consumption of many health-harming substances.

9. If your oil (or food cooked in oil) starts smoking, throw it out and start over.

10. Use the salt of the earth or sea—Himalayan crystal or Celtic sea salt—sparingly.

11. Can the soda—all kinds.

You can combine this phase of *The Life Force Diet* with the next one (found in Chapter 5) or you can take a week, two weeks, or even a month to gradually eliminate the 3Ps from your diet, if that is easier for you. Choose what works best for your personality and lifestyle, and then stick with it. Once you have weaned the three Ps out of your diet, stick with it for at least three weeks so that you can begin to feel the wonderful health benefits and the return of energy. I think you'll agree: It's miraculous!

Avoid health-harming junk. Commit to this for the three-week plan, and after that you'll probably realize you no longer want junk food. If you're choosing the life force diet as a permanent lifestyle change, don't worry about the occasional treat. Besides, over time, you'll discover that when you "treat" yourself with junk foods, your body doesn't feel like it has been "treated" well at all.

5

Week Two—Start with the Silver

*"One of the very nicest things about life is the
way we must regularly stop whatever it is we
are doing and devote our attention to eating."*

—Luciano Pavarotti

BETTER known for his classical singing than for his philosophies on food, Luciano Pavarotti made the above declaration about eating in his autobiography, and I couldn't agree more. Yet most people never devote their attention to eating. And somehow too many people have the ludicrous idea that eating healthily means sacrificing taste. That's a dangerous myth that I hope to destroy. Some of the healthiest foods are among the most delicious.

Last week you eliminated or greatly reduced many harmful substances in your diet. That allowed your body to improve its ability to detoxify substances that interfere or impede natural enzyme functions. It's critical that we tackled this step first to eliminate obstacles that may prevent the natural performance of enzymes and the countless biochemical processes they are involved in. During, the second week of the program we'll set the stage for optimal health by providing the essential nutrients that ensure the proper functioning of life force enzymes. By ramping up the macronutrients, vitamins, minerals, and phytonutrients (we'll discuss phytonutrients momentarily), you'll kick-start your body's natural enzyme processes. And next week we'll add plentiful amounts of enzyme-rich foods to give your internal enzymes a serious boost. By working in this systematic fashion, your body is better able to perform its trillions of functions, thereby improving your weight, immunity to illness, and even its regenerative powers.

Keep in mind that Life Force Silver Foods are excellent and delicious foods in their own right and not simply substitutions for unhealthy options. And don't worry if you're not sure what to do with these foods; I'll provide lots of suggestions throughout this chapter, along with delicious recipes incorporating both Life Force Silver and Gold Foods in Chapter 9.

When you start with the Silver, you'll begin to make better and healthier dietary choices. Life Force Silver Foods include wild salmon, sweet potatoes, lentils, beans, wild rice, and most vegetables, to name a few. These delicious, health-building foods are packed with nutrients and are also loaded with many phytonutrients as well—both of which help prevent and fight disease, while giving you greater energy and vitality.

Let me start by introducing you to a sampling of the Life Force Silver Foods.

Life Force Silver Foods	
Grains, Breads, Cereals, Pastas	
Enjoy breads, cereals, and pastas made with any of the following grains:	
Amaranth	Buckwheat flour
Arrowroot flour	Chickpea flour
Barley	Coconut flour
Barley flour	Kamut
Brown rice	Kamut flour
Brown rice flour	Millet
Buckwheat	Oat flour

Oats

Quinoa

Spelt

Spelt flour

Sprouted grains

Tapioca flour

Wild rice

Legumes (Beans)

Aduki beans

Black beans

Black-eyed peas

Garbanzo beans (chickpeas)

Kidney beans

Lentils

Lima beans

Navy beans

Pinto beans

Romano beans

Other types of beans

Beverages

Black tea

Green tea

Herbal tea (licorice, ginger,
chamomile, peppermint, etc.)

Herbal coffee substitutes made
from roasted dandelion or
chicory

Fish*

Herring

Lake Trout

Mackerel

Sardines

Wild salmon

Vegetables

Asparagus

Bamboo Shoots

Beetroot

Broccoli

Brussels sprouts

Cabbage (purple or green)

Carrots (cooked)

Cauliflower

Celery

Celery root (celeriac)

Collard greens

Corn (fresh)

Dandelion greens

Eggplant

Fennel

Garlic

Ginger

Green beans

Green peppers

Hot peppers / chilies

Jerusalem artichoke

Kale

Continued on page 112

Continued from page III

Life Force Silver Foods	
Vegetables	
Leeks	Spices (fresh or non-irradiated,
Mushrooms	organic, dried spices)
Olives	Spinach
Onions	Squash
Peas	Sweet potato
Pumpkin	Tomatoes
Red peppers	Water chestnuts
Seaweed	Yellow or orange peppers
Shallots	Zucchini

Any of the Life Force Gold Foods that have been cooked—you'll find them listed in the next chapter.

* While there are many other types of fish that contain high amounts of Omega-3 fatty acids, the Life Force Silver selections typically contain fewer toxins and heavy metals than others.

What separates a Life Force Silver Food from a Gold Food? Simple—both are nutritional powerhouses, but Life Force Silver Foods are cooked. Don't panic that you'll be grazing on grass or crunching carrot sticks all day. I assure you that you'll be surprised at how great both Life Force Gold and Silver Foods taste. In the next chapter we'll explore lots of quick, delicious, and even many gourmet ways to get more Life Force Gold Foods into your diet.

The life force diet is packed with nutrition and flavour, so it wouldn't be complete without the staples, sweeteners, and condiments that complement the natural flavours of life force silver and gold foods. By now, you've already eliminated the many unhealthy options of these foods in your fridge and pantry. I've included the following table to help you get started restocking with healthier options. Of course, it's impossible to create an exhaustive list, especially as new options are coming onto the market all the time. Use your best judgment based on the new principles you've learned: Avoid foods that are overly refined and/or that contain colours; preservatives; excessive, refined, or synthetic sweeteners; trans or hydrogenated fats; or other suspect ingredients. Yes, that means reading the labels on foods! It may feel difficult at first, but you'll be surprised how quickly this becomes easy for you.

Staples, Sweeteners, and Condiments	
Condiments	
Fruit jams (made from 100% fruit and which do not contain added sugars)	Mustard
	Nama shoyu
	Pickled Ginger
Ketchup	Tamari (alternative to soy sauce)
Meat and Eggs*	
Beef	Eggs
Bison/Buffalo	Lamb
Chicken	Turkey
Duck	
Soy Products**	
Cheonggukjang	Natto
Chunjang	Pickled Tofu
Doenjang	Tauchu
Doubanjiang	Tempeh
Gochujang	Tofu
Miso	
Sweeteners	
Agave nectar	Molasses (natural varieties that
Barley malt syrup	are made without chemical
Brown rice syrup	extracts)
Honey, unpasteurized	Stevia rebaudiana (often just
Maple syrup (100% pure, preferably "Number 3" since it is less refined)	called "stevia")

Continued on page 114

Continued from page 113

Staples, Sweeteners, and Condiments	
Vinegars***	
Apple cider vinegar	Red wine vinegar
Balsamic vinegar (with naturally	Rice wine vinegar
occurring sulfites only)	White wine vinegar

*Choose organic lean cuts of meat only. Duck tends to be high in fat and should be eaten in modest amounts only. White meat from chicken and turkey is a superior option to red meat.

** Be sure to read "The Pros and Cons of Soybeans" on page 124" to help you decide whether soy products are right for you.

*** If you choose flavoured vinegars, be sure they are in a base of one of the vinegar types on this list, otherwise they are generally just white vinegar with herbs or fruit added and should be avoided.

Stock Your Life Force Kitchen

Now that your cupboards and fridge are free from junk foods and other life force destroyers, it's time to replenish them with delicious, nutritious Life Force Silver Foods, like those in the chart above. Now is the time to pick your favourite five veggies from the list above as well as two you don't usually buy or maybe haven't tried and add them to your grocery list.

Instead of passing by the fresh herbs in your grocery story, add a couple to your order. Choose two of the above grains and beans from the Life Force Silver Foods list. Most grocery stores now offer a variety of options for pasta such as spelt pasta or brown rice pasta. Choose these excellent options instead of white or wheat pasta. If you choose canned beans, make sure they are EDTA-free since you don't want to be ingesting preservatives on the life force diet.

Also stock your pantry with coconut milk (the full-fat kind, not the low-fat version since most of the health benefits are in the fatty part of the milk), unpasteurized honey, extra virgin and cold-pressed olive oil, or coconut oil. The latter is typically found in a large jar and is solid at room temperature. While the latter two foods are Life

Force Gold Foods, you'll probably want to add them to your grocery order immediately since they make excellent cooking oils for many of the foods you'll be eating this week.

If you're eating meat on the life force diet, now is the time to visit your local butcher to locate lean, organic cuts of meat as a complement to your meals. Remember that meat and fish should not be the focal point of our meals. You may want to add wild salmon or other fish listed above to your grocery order as well.

If you haven't visited your local natural foods store (or it it's been a while), now is the time to do so. While you're there, choose healthier versions of your favourite staples, sweeteners, and condiments, such as those listed above. While we're discussing condiments, were you surprised to see ketchup on the list? You can enjoy condiments like ketchup as long as you choose brands that are devoid of preservatives, colours, synthetic sweeteners or high fructose corn syrup, and other additives (the same goes for all condiments and packaged foods). They should be minimally but naturally sweetened and low in sodium. Another option for healthier condiments is to make them at home, which is usually easier than you think!

Remember that you don't have to give up all carbohydrates on the life force diet either. Your body needs them as a source of energy, but they just have to come from the right source. Select pastas and breads made from whole grain kamut, spelt, or brown rice flour (or another type from the chart above). You can also choose breads, wraps, or pasta made with sprouted grains, since they are whole grains that are predigested during the sprouting process. You'll soon discover some new favourite, delicious carbs.

Ignite Your Life Force

STEP 12 Eat Lots of Life Force Silver Foods

This week as you start the second week of the life force diet you should be eating no more than 15 percent of your diet as animal protein (meat, poultry, fish, or eggs). The remainder of your diet should comprise Life Force Silver Foods like those listed in the earlier chart. It's easier than you think to eat plentiful amounts of Life Force Silver Foods. If you're having trouble finding ways to enjoy them, I've provided many breakfast, snack, salad, and other life force suggestions in the recipe section at the back of this book.

Now that you've learned about many of the critical nutrients and enzymes needed for optimum health, you may be wondering why the life force diet includes any cooked food at all. I've included them for a few reasons.

First, very few of us would really be satisfied with a diet made up entirely of uncooked foods. By next week (and I hope thereafter) you'll be eating 15 percent animal protein (if you choose to eat meat during the program), 35 percent Life Force Silver Foods, and 50 percent Life Force Gold Foods. If you're opting to go vegetarian throughout the program, you'll be eating 50 percent Life Force Silver Foods and 50 percent Life Force Gold Foods. Let's face it: Cooked food tastes good. And, if you live in a colder climate, you probably couldn't bear the thought of eating something cold when you come in from an icy winter day. But don't worry, in the next chapter I'll provide easy ways to increase the amount of enzyme-rich food in your diet even when it's cold outside.

Second, there are many important nutrients in Life Force Silver Foods. Most Life Force Silver Foods are packed with many vitamins, minerals, amino acids, complex carbohydrates, and essential fatty acids, making them nutritional powerhouses that are an important part of your diet. While most nutrients are better absorbed from uncooked foods, a few phytonutrients like lycopene found in tomatoes are actually better absorbed by your body once foods containing them have been cooked. But, I'm getting ahead of myself. We'll discuss phytonutrients momentarily.

Third, in addition to their high amounts of important nutrients, Life Force Silver and Gold Foods contain a whole variety of plant nutrients (phytonutrients) such as sulforaphane, lipoic acid, catechins, and more. Different foods contain different disease-fighting phytonutrients. You don't have to memorize their names or learn which foods contain these disease-fighting compounds. By simply eating a variety of Life Force Silver Foods that will comprise 50 percent of all the foods you eat in a day, you'll be getting plentiful amounts of these life force builders. Let's explore some of the phytonutrients found in Life Force Silver and Gold Foods and their many miracle healing properties so you'll better understand why you'd want to include them in your diet.

Ignite Your Life Force

> ### STEP 13 Choose Your Veggies
> Choose five of your favourite vegetables as well as two that you don't normally buy or haven't tried and add them to your grocery order this week. And be sure they don't just sit in your refrigerator. Sauté, steam, bake, or stir-fry them as part of your lunches and dinners.

Micronutrients—Natural Life Force Phytonutrients

Most of us have heard that fruits and vegetables have been shown to lower cholesterol and blood pressure (when it is high), reduce the risk of developing cataracts and macular degeneration leading to vision loss, balance blood sugar levels, balance weight, improve bowel regularity and colon health, as well as guard against cancer. Not only does their incredible array of macronutrients, vitamins, and minerals play a role in their healing powers, so do nutrients known as phytonutrients and enzymes. We discussed the importance of enzymes in Chapter 2 and I share more information about how to obtain them in the next chapter. But first let's explore phytonutrients. Once you know about their health marvels, I'm sure you'll agree that these are foods you'll definitely want in your diet.

There are about 2000 known phytonutrients and many others are being discovered all the time. And, you guessed it, they're found in fruit, vegetables, herbs, spices, nuts, sprouts, and seeds that comprise the Life Force Gold and Silver Foods. A single fruit or vegetable may contain more than 100 types of healing phytonutrients that basically make up the immune system of the plant. Once eaten, they impart their miraculous healing abilities inside your body. The thousands of phytonutrients are categorized into families, including carotenoids, catechins, flavonoids, lipoic acid, phytoestrogens, polyphenols, sulfurophane, and others. Let's explore the phytonutrient families and find out how you can include more of them in your diet.

Anthocyanins

These natural, health-boosting substances give certain fruits their purple to reddish colour. Not only does research show that anthocyanins have the capacity to boost short-term memory by 100 percent in just eight weeks, they also stimulate the burning of stored fat in the body to be used as fuel. A group of laboratory animals fed a high-fat diet along with anthocyanins gained 24 percent less weight than their counterparts fed only the fatty diet, according to research published in *The Journal of Agricultural and Food Chemistry*.[1] Anthocyanins are found in dark purple or red grapes, cherries, and berries, including blueberries, blackberries, raspberries, and strawberries.

Carotenoids

Carotenoids are the yellow, orange, and red pigments found in foods like carrots, sweet potatoes, apricots, mangoes, pumpkin, tomatoes, papaya, peaches, and other similarly coloured foods. Dark green vegetables like broccoli and leafy greens also contain high amounts of carotenoids. You may have heard about beta-carotene, lutein, and lycopene, all of which are specific types of carotenoids. Not only do these nutrients help strengthen our eyesight and boost our immunity to disease, they are powerful antioxidants that help ward off cancer and protect against the effects of aging. Studies at Harvard University of more than 124,000 people showed a 32 percent reduction in risk of lung cancer in people who consumed a variety of carotenoid-rich foods as part of their regular diet.[2] Another study of women who had completed treatment for early stage breast cancer conducted by researchers at Women's Healthy Eating and Living (WHEL) found that women with the highest blood concentrations of carotenoids had the least likelihood of cancer recurrence.[3]

Catechins

The full name for these natural plant compounds is catechin polyphenols. They activate fat-burning genes in abdominal fat cells to assist with weight loss, and belly fat loss in particular. According to research at Tufts University, catechins increase abdominal fat loss by 77 percent and double total weight loss. As if that wasn't enough reason for most of us to include foods high in catechins like green and black tea and apples in our diet, catechins also improve your body's ability to use insulin secreted by your pancreas, which prevents blood sugar spikes and crashes involved in plummeting energy levels, cravings, depression, and mood swings.

Scientists have even discovered that epigallocatechin gallate (or EGCG for short), a particular type of catechin, is 200 times more powerful at eliminating free radicals that damage the skin than vitamin E.[4]

Flavonoids

This group of phytonutrients is showing huge promise as miracle healing substances. Found in berries, cherries, currants, pomegranates, red and purple grapes, red onions, tomatoes, bell peppers, apple (skin), and walnuts, flavonoids interfere with stages of the development of cancer cells, thereby preventing their ability to keep multiplying. Ellagic acid also encourages a healthy rate of a natural process in the body called apoptosis. Apoptosis is the body's way of ensuring damaged cells are killed so they cannot harm the body. A healthy rate of apoptosis essentially ensures cancer cells are killed by the body. Ellagic acid also helps stimulate the detoxification enzymes in the liver, thereby helping the liver to eliminate environmental toxins, excess hormones, and food toxins, and perform its hundreds of important functions normally.

The flavonoid resveratrol has been getting a tremendous amount of media exposure lately, due to its powerful ability to protect the brain from damage. Dr. Egemen Savaskan and colleagues at the University of Basel in Switzerland discovered resveratrol in grapes. This compound may even help protect the brain against Alzheimer's disease. They found that resveratrol protected brain cells from plaque formation linked to the disease by mopping up free radicals. Grapes are currently the best known source of this potent healing substance. While red wine is a good source of resveratrol, its alcohol content can be damaging to brain cells and the liver.

Another group of flavonoids called proanthocyanins have demonstrated the unique capacity to protect both the fatty and non-fatty parts of the brain against damage from some environmental toxins. They appear to work by decreasing free radical activity within and between brain cells.[5] Blueberries have some of the highest concentrations of these potent antioxidants.

Lipoic Acid

Lipoic acid is a powerful antioxidant that has the ability to mop up free radicals linked to aging and disease. Additionally, within cells, it has the ability to increase the production of leptin, which appears to stifle the production of the chemical ghrelin linked to increased appetite. In other words, lipoic acid can help turn off hunger pangs.

Women taking lipoic acid in scientific studies were found to have lost 5 percent of their body weight within six months.[6] Lipoic acid has also been shown to power up the energy centres of the cells, called mitochondria, helping them to work more effectively. That means increased energy for you! Researchers at the University of California at Berkeley found that lipoic acid had the ability to double energy levels in their subjects. Lipoic acid is found in plentiful amounts in Life Force Silver Foods like dark leafy greens. Kale, Swiss chard, collard greens, and spinach are all good sources.

Phytoestrogens

Phytoestrogens are plant estrogens, which are natural plant hormones. They play an important role in helping to regulate hormones in the body, thereby reducing the likelihood of hormone-related cancers like breast and prostate cancer, as well as assisting with maintaining a healthy hormone balance during perimenopause (up to a decade prior to menopause) and menopause. Phytoestrogens are naturally found in seeds, grains, some fruits and vegetables, and in higher quantities in soy foods like soymilk, tofu, etc. We'll discuss more about the pros and cons of soy later in this chapter.

Polyphenols

Found in nuts, berries, and tea, polyphenols are powerful antioxidants with anti-inflammatory properties. Additionally, they are antiallergenic, meaning that they help reduce the biochemical processes that are linked to allergic reactions.

Sulfuraphane

The phytochemical sulfurophane lowers blood levels of cancer-stimulating estrogens in the blood in as few as five days, according to the American Institute for Cancer Research. Sulfurophane also halts the growth of cancer cells on contact. For those readers looking to lose weight, this powerful phytochemical can increase weight loss by as much as 22 percent, according to research at Nashville's Vanderbilt Medical Center.[7] It works by releasing trapped toxins that slow metabolism and increase fat storage within fat cells. Sulfurophane is found in the Life Force Silver Foods: broccoli, cabbage, Brussels sprouts, cauliflower, bok choy, and other cruciferous vegetables, as in well as dark leafy greens.

Terpenes

Found in citrus fruits like lemons, limes, oranges, and grapefruits, there are numerous terpenes that offer health benefits, including limonoids. There are about 40 types of limonoids. Research shows that they have powerful anti-cancer activity and significantly improve the liver's ability to eliminate toxins we've inhaled or ingested, including cancer-causing agents.

While there are thousands of phytonutrients with as many healing properties, they share a common role as nature's miracle healers. Not only do they help prevent countless diseases and reverse many illnesses, they also strengthen immunity, boost energy, improve cellular functioning, slow the aging process, and help restore healthy and balanced weight.

Getting a broad spectrum of phytonutrients is part of the key to maximize great health. So how do you know if you're getting a wide range of phytonutrients? Simple. Eat a wide variety of fruits and vegetables and make a conscious effort to get a whole range of colours every day. If you eat yellow-orange, red, green, and bluish purple fruits and vegetables every day, you can feel confident that you've ingested hundreds of phytonutrients that will not only impart their disease-prevention powers, but also increase your sense of well-being. For example, if in a day you drink a glass of water with fresh lemon juice, and eat a plate full of salad greens topped with strawberries, enjoy roasted sweet potatoes, along with a blueberry-banana/almond milk smoothie (along with whatever else you may eat that day), you'll have covered all the colours of the phytonutrient rainbow.

Ignite Your Life Force

STEP 14 Ramp Up Your Phytonutrients

Eat yellow-orange, red, green, and bluish-purple fruits and vegetables every day starting this week. That could include carrots, red peppers, salad greens, and blueberries to cover the full spectrum of foods. Or you could have sweet potatoes, strawberries, asparagus, and cherries. These foods can be eaten at any meal. It really doesn't matter whether you have them at breakfast, lunch, dinner, for snacks, or a combination of all of the above. In a couple of weeks you can relax these efforts a bit while still trying to get a wide variety of colour in your daily diet. But for the next two weeks be sure to get a full spectrum of colourful fruits and vegetables into your diet.

Beans, Beans, the Magical Health Food

Beans are the most underappreciated foods, yet they offer an incredible assortment of nutrients, are a high-quality protein, a "good carb," and an excellent source of fibre. Most types of beans contain high levels of vitamins B1 and B6 and folate, which are helpful for handling stress, improving energy production, maintaining proper brain cell functioning, balancing moods, helping to keep the skin, muscles, liver, and other organs in excellent condition, and much more. Kidney beans are high in the mineral manganese, which your body requires to make an important enzyme called "superoxide dismutase" or "SOD" for short. SOD disarms free radicals produced in the energy centres of your body's cells, thereby increasing energy production and lessening free radical damage that is linked to aging and disease. Some beans like black-eyed peas even enhance the body's ability to make DNA.

Because beans are high in fibre, they help to stabilize blood sugar levels for hours, making you less vulnerable to energy or mood crashes and cravings. Their high fibre content also helps you feel full for hours, making them an excellent health food if you're trying to lose weight.

It's easy to add kidney beans, aduki beans, mung beans, pinto beans, black-eyed peas, black beans, lima beans, lentils, black beans, garbanzo beans (chickpeas), navy beans, or other beans to your diet to reap their many health rewards; they are one of my favourite Life Force Silver Foods!

Ignite Your Life Force

> **STEP 15 Eat More Beans**
>
> Try to get at least ½ cup of cooked beans or uncooked bean sprouts (more on this topic in the next chapter) into your daily diet. With so many to choose from, you'll be surprised how easy it actually is. You can eat black beans or kidney beans in chili, add cooked garbanzo beans to a salad, enjoy lentils in a soup or stew, or purée pinto beans with some sautéed onions and a dash of Celtic sea salt for delicious un-fried "refried beans." You can add some seasonings and blend beans to make a paté, sandwich spread, or dip. Check out the hummus recipe at the back of this book for a delicious sandwich spread or veggie dip. You can cook dried beans almost effortlessly by adding beans and water to a slow cooker and cooking on low overnight. The beans will be ready to add to your favourite recipe by morning. If you're pressed for time, just open a can of EDTA-free beans, rinse thoroughly and add to your favourite recipe, toss on a salad, or add to a soup or stew.

The Pros and Cons of Soybeans

Almost everybody these days is confused about soy. One publication touts soy's incredible health properties and phytonutrients, while another indicates that soy is harmful to your health. What's a person to believe? When it comes to soy, I think it's important to weigh several factors before deciding if soy is right or wrong for your body, particularly since the issues may be different for different people's bodies.

Soybeans have been eaten as part of Asian diets for thousands of year. However, most writers overstate the role of soy in the Asian diet, claiming that Asians eat far more soy products than they actually do. In more recent years, large corporations began growing and harvesting soybean crops for large-scale food manufacturing. In doing so, many companies have adopted unsustainable practices such as using genetically modified soybeans, spraying plants with harmful pesticides, and even chopping down precious rainforest areas to maximize their profits. These types of practices not only cause widespread planetary destruction, they pose a threat to the health of people as well. The use of toxic pesticides, many of which are known neurotoxins—they damage the brain and nervous system—is a dangerous practice no matter the food crop being sprayed. As for genetically modified (GM) foods, research is increasingly linking their consumption to serious health concerns—again, whether the crop is soy, wheat, corn, canola, or any other type. Inadequate long-term research has been conducted on the effects of consuming GM foods; however, since 75 percent of foods found in your grocery store have been genetically modified, I truly believe that we are in the midst of a wide-scale experiment. And the effects may be seen in the skyrocketing incidence of disease. While there are certainly other factors at play with the disease statistics we are experiencing at this time in our history, over time I am confident that genetically modified foods, including GM soy and soy products, are at least playing a role in our rapidly increasing rates of heart disease, diabetes, arthritis, and cancer, as well as many other illnesses.

Another part of the love-hate relationship with soy is its high phytoestrogen content. Phytoestrogens are natural plant hormones that mimic estrogen in our bodies. For some people these estrogens may help balance their hormones, particularly during the menopausal years for women who may be deficient in estrogens. However, these estrogens may throw off the hormonal balance for other people. Phytoestrogens attach to estrogen receptor sites in the body, blocking the ability of xenoestrogens to bind to these sites. Xenoestrogens are chemical estrogen mimickers that are found in many foods, plastic substances, and household items and are known to cause serious hormonal imbalances. You may have heard about bisphenol A (BPA) and its worrisome prevalence in the manufacture of plastic water and beverage bottles, as well as in other consumer products. BPA is just one type of damaging xenoestrogen to which we are exposed. Most xenoestrogens are roughly 100 times stronger than human estrogens. The natural estrogen found in soy is extremely mild and closer to human estrogen than xenoestrogens. For many people, the addition of phytoestrogens (plant estrogen) found in soy can be beneficial, both to block xenoestrogens and also to help balance potentially low levels of human estrogens. But any amount of phytoestrogen can be too much in someone with already excessively high levels.

People with low thyroid functioning also need to limit their soy consumption since soy contains substances called goitrogens which can slow the production and/or release of thyroid hormones in the body. Most people with hypothyroidism, as this common condition is called, can tolerate up to about 1 cup of organic soy milk daily without negative consequences on hormone production. But it's best to consult with your doctor or natural health practitioner if you have any concerns about eating soy products.

Fermented soy products are actually the easiest to digest and the best tolerated by people. Traditional Asian diets typically contain more fermented soy products like miso than non-fermented forms of soy. Some fermented soy products include tamari, pickled tofu, natto, tempeh, cheonggukjang, chunjang, doenjang, doubanjiang, gochujang, and tauchu. Fermented soy products like these are acceptable on the life force diet, as is unsweetened soy milk when drunk in moderation only (1 to 2 cups daily). The latter should be made from only non-genetically modified, unsprayed, sustainably harvested organic soybeans, free of sugar, artificial sweeteners, or other additives.

How to Satisfy Your Cravings on the Life Force Diet

Okay, who hasn't experienced the overwhelming desire to eat something specific, whether it be chocolate, potato chips, a burger, or some other food? We've all experienced cravings, but we should be careful about the way in which we satisfy them. By understanding what your body is actually deficient in (assuming it is a physical, not an emotional food craving) you can get to the root cause of the cravings, and eventually kick them all together.

There are numerous possible meanings of cravings, depending on the type of craving and your eating habits. Before you satisfy cravings, drink a tall glass of pure water. Quite often we misinterpret our body's signal for thirst as a signal of hunger. By drinking a tall glass of water first, you may be giving your body exactly what it wants and alleviate craving. Some experts estimate that up to 80 percent of the population is chronically dehydrated, so start with water before you try to decipher your cravings.

Ignite Your Life Force

STEP 16 Curb Cravings

If you experience cravings, it may be your body's attempt to tell you that you're dehydrated. At the first sign of a craving, drink a tall glass of pure water. If after about a half an hour you are still experiencing a food craving, choose a healthy snack to help balance your blood sugar levels, since low blood sugar may be contributing

> to your cravings. That's typically enough to eliminate most cravings. Throughout this week and next, you'll be eating more nutrient-rich food and that will help to quell any nutrient deficiencies that are masquerading as cravings. If you're still suffering from cravings by the end of this week, be sure to review the following section to see what nutrients you may need.

If you're still craving other foods, you may also be deficient in particular nutrients. For example:

Chocolate—If you crave chocolate, it doesn't mean your body has a chocolate deficiency, although I think most people would prefer that. Chocolate is high in magnesium. Cravings for it often indicate that your body is deficient in magnesium, which is a common deficiency. If you're going to eat chocolate, choose organic cocoa and mix it into a healthy smoothie, or eat a small amount of dark chocolate. Because that is unlikely enough to deal with a magnesium deficiency, it's also important to eat other foods high in magnesium, such as nuts, seeds, fish, and leafy greens.

Sweets—If you crave sweets you may be experiencing blood sugar fluctuations. When your blood sugar drops, your body may be trying to get you to give it more fuel to keep your blood sugar levels stable. If this is a chronic occurrence you may have hypoglycemia, which simply means low blood sugar. Whether your sugar cravings are sporadic or chronic, it is important to choose the right type of food to bring your body back into balance. Giving in to cookies, cakes, candies, or other refined sweets will only make the problem worse and cause a blood sugar roller coaster that leads to more cravings. Instead, choose a piece of fruit when you're craving sweets. In the interim, add more high-fibre foods like beans and legumes, and complex carbohydrates like whole grains to give you the fuel you need without the blood sugar spikes. If you're really struggling with sugar cravings, you may also wish to supplement with the mineral chromium since it helps to regulate blood sugar levels and ward off cravings.

Salty Foods—Cravings for salty foods like popcorn or chips often indicate stress hormone fluctuations in the body. Getting on top of the stress in your life is step one. The adrenal glands help your body cope with stress and, in our fast-paced, hectic lives, tend to become worn out, especially from stress-hormone production. Try meditation, breathing exercises, or other stress management techniques. Research at the University of Utah in Salt Lake City showed that people who take a break to breathe deeply or meditate before reaching for salty snacks reduced their stress hormones by 25 percent and cut the bingeing in half.

If your adrenal glands are worn out, you can also support them with a high-quality B-complex vitamin, with extra pantothenic acid (that's vitamin B-5) and vitamin C. Eating more leafy greens helps to supply your body with minerals that support the adrenal glands, especially potassium.

Red Meat—Not surprisingly, cravings for red meat usually indicate an iron deficiency. Often people crave burgers or steaks. Women of menstruation age are especially vulnerable to iron deficiencies. Eat more iron-rich beans and legumes, unsulphured prunes, figs, and other dried fruits. If you are eating meat on the life force diet, you can also choose lean, organic red meat like beef or bison as a source of iron. Just remember to keep meat consumption to within 15 percent of your total daily diet. Vitamin C helps with the absorption of iron, so take vitamin C alongside your iron-rich foods. Alternatively, eat citrus, red peppers, tomatoes, or berries which are high in vitamin C with your iron-rich foods.

Cheese—Cravings for cheese or pizza often indicate a fatty acid deficiency, which is common in most people. Eat foods such as raw walnuts, wild salmon, flax oil; add ground flaxseeds to your diet. Supplement with a high-quality supplement that includes the beneficial fats, especially Omega 3s. It should contain both EPA and DHA. Two to three servings of fish such as wild salmon or a small handful of raw walnuts or 2 tablespoons of ground flaxseeds in a smoothie will often cut out cheese cravings altogether.

Snacky—If you often feel snacky, sometimes for sweets, sometimes for salty foods, it can mean you're not eating a well-balanced diet and may be missing a variety of nutrients. Get started with weeks one and two of the life force diet right away, cutting out the junk and adding more delicious, healthful foods. Also, add a good multivitamin and mineral to your day.

Reaching for junk foods at the onset of cravings will only satisfy them temporarily. Making dietary changes that address deficiencies or imbalances can help eliminate them altogether.

Ignite Your Life Force

> **STEP 17** Snack Your Way to Stronger Life Force
>
> It's important to eat every two to three hours to regulate blood sugar levels and control cravings. It's easy to do. Simply snack between meals. Munch on celery sticks with almond butter, eat veggies with hummus (see recipe in Chapter 9), or eat a piece of fruit. By snacking between meals, you'll balance your blood sugar, which in turn helps to balance your energy levels, moods, and speed weight loss if you're overweight.

Summary of Week Two of the Life Force Diet

1. Eat lots of Life Force Silver Foods. If you're eating meat, poultry, or fish it should comprise 15 percent of your daily diet at most.

2. Choose a variety of veggies. Select at least five of your favourites and two that you don't normally eat every day.

3. Ramp up your phytonutrients by eating yellow-orange, red, green, and bluish-purple produce daily to ensure you're getting a wide variety.

4. Eat more beans—1/2 cup minimum daily.

5. Curb cravings. Counter cravings by drinking a glass of water at the first sign of a craving. Wait half an hour. If that doesn't work, eat a piece of fruit if you're craving something sweet, and address other likely causes of your cravings from the list in pages 128-130. If you're still suffering from cravings, take a chromium supplement to help keep blood sugar balanced.

6. Snack your way to stronger life force. Make sure you're eating something healthy every two to three hours to balance your blood sugar levels.

7. Start taking one to two capsules of a full-spectrum enzyme supplement with every meal to assist with digestion and to ensure you're assimilating the many nutrients found in the foods you're eating. See Chapter 7 for more information on choosing a high-quality enzyme supplement.

Introducing the Sensational Life Force Silver Foods

There are many excellent Life Force Silver Foods. Don't worry if you're not familiar with them all. I've included nutritional information for each, along with suggestions on how to use some of them. Also, consult the recipes in Chapter 9 for more delicious food ideas.

Asparagus—An excellent source of nutrients like vitamin K and folate, asparagus also contains good amounts of vitamins C, A, B1, B2, niacin, B6, manganese, potassium, magnesium, and selenium, not to mention that it is delicious, particularly steamed and topped with a bit of my flax butter (see Michelle's Better Butter recipe on page 230). Its high-folate content makes it a particularly good food for pregnant women. I also enjoy steamed or roasted asparagus atop a bed of leafy greens and completed with a citrus dressing such as my Life Force Salad Dressing (see page 245).

Beets—Recommended by holistic health professionals to help purify the blood and cleanse the liver, beets are also high in nutrients such as folate, manganese, potassium, and vitamin C. In their uncooked state, beets also contain an important compound called betaine, which research has shown reduces several compounds linked to inflammation in the body. In other words, it's a great anti-inflammatory food that helps protect us from the effects of aging and disease. The phytonutrient that gives beets their rich purplish-red hue is a potent cancer fighter. What's more, the fibre found in beets seems to increase the body's special immune compounds that are responsible for detecting and removing abnormal cells before they can become cancerous. Beets are one of Nature's miracles in the prevention of cancer. They can be eaten raw (grated), steamed, boiled (although many nutrients are lost in the cooking water), or added to soups and stews. I love steamed beets tossed with a little of Michelle's Better Butter and Celtic sea salt. Remember: The anti-cancer properties of beets lessen with heat! So it's always a great idea to enjoy a little grated beetroot on your salads.

Black Beans—Because black beans are high in fibre, they help to stabilize blood sugar levels and escort toxins from the colon. That may be part of the reason why they help to prevent cancer. As food is digested, potential carcinogens from insecticides or processing can become more concentrated. The fibre in black beans can bind to these carcinogens and other toxins to eliminate them from the body. With over 6 grams of fibre per ½ cup serving, black beans are a must as part of the life force diet. Black beans also lower cholesterol levels to help reduce the risk of diabetes, heart attack, and stroke. Plus, eating a high-fibre diet helps to protect against colon/rectal cancer.

Broccoli—In addition to containing plentiful amounts of nutrients such as vitamins A, B2, B6, C, K, folate, manganese, potassium, magnesium, and many others, this cruciferous vegetable is a superb cancer-fighter. Thanks to the phytonutrients sulfurophane and the indoles, broccoli is a potent weapon against this serious disease. Sulfurophane protects against colon cancer and helps the liver to detoxify harmful chemicals, including those that may be carcinogens. In research, the indoles appear to deactivate estrogens that promote tumour growth, such as is found in breast cancer. At the same time, indoles seem to encourage the production of particular types of estrogens that fight cancer. I enjoy steamed broccoli tossed in some finely minced fresh garlic, a touch of Michelle's Better Butter, and some freshly squeezed lemon juice. Contrary to common belief, there are many great ways to enjoy broccoli, and it is a worthy addition to your diet.

Brown Rice—High in fibre and complex carbohydrates, brown rice helps to keep your blood sugar levels (and therefore, energy, moods, and weight) stable while still providing your body with energy for fuel. Its high-fibre content also helps reduce your risk of colon cancer or other bowel disorders. Because it is naturally gluten-free, it is an excellent grain for those suffering from celiac disease or anyone suffering from an inflammatory disorder (since gluten may be linked to inflammation in the body). Don't worry if you're not a huge fan of brown rice—I'm not!—but I've included a delicious recipe for Pineapple Basil Rice (see page 250) that will turn any brown rice hater into a lover of this nutritious food. I usually recommend adding more water and overcooking brown rice slightly to help make it more easily digestible.

Carrots—Not only an incredibly versatile vegetable, carrots are also packed with nutrition, particularly beta carotene. A single raw carrot contains 13,500 IU of this potent antioxidant. If you're not sure what that means ... it means a whole lot of free radical fighting ability to protect against cellular damage, premature aging, cataracts, and even cancer. Plus, carrots are rich in fibre, including a particular type that is effective at reducing cholesterol. According to scientists at the United States Department of Agriculture, eating two carrots daily may reduce total cholesterol levels by 20 percent in those people with elevated levels.[8]

Cauliflower—Did you know that cauliflower eaters have lower rates of cancer than people who don't indulge in this vegetable or other cruciferous vegetables such as broccoli and Brussels sprouts? That's because cauliflower, like other cruciferous vegetables, contains sulforaphane. According to researchers at Johns Hopkins University School of Medicine, this potent phytonutrient stimulates the body's production of cancer-fighting enzymes.[9] Cauliflower also packs a sizable dose of vitamin C, potassium, fibre, and other important vitamins and minerals.

Celery (and Celery Seeds)—This frequently overlooked vegetable deserves its rightful place in the Life Force Silver Foods or Life Force Gold Foods if you eat it in its uncooked form. Both celery and its seeds contain at least 20 anti-pain and anti-inflammatory compounds, making it an anti-aging miracle food. Modern theories of aging propose that inflammation in the body is largely responsible for premature aging and many of its signs, including wrinkling, sagging skin, and more. Celery and celery seeds are particularly great for anyone suffering from pain disorders such as arthritis and fibromyalgia. Additionally, Traditional Chinese Medicine doctors have used celery to treat high blood pressure for thousands of years. Most North American medical doctors tell patients to avoid celery due to its high sodium content. However, researchers at the University of Chicago have sided with the Chinese practitioners after identifying a potent phytonutrient called 3-butylphthalide, which they demonstrated reduces blood pressure in laboratory rats by relaxing the smooth muscle lining of the blood vessels, thereby allowing the blood to flow more freely throughout the blood vessels. When fed the equivalent amount of phthalide to that which is found in four stalks of celery for an average human, the rats experienced a 13 percent drop in blood pressure and a 7 percent drop in cholesterol levels.[10]

Chickpeas (Garbanzo Beans)—Like most legumes, chickpeas are packed with protein, fibre, minerals like molybdenum, manganese, and iron, as well as vitamins such as folate (vitamin B9). Their high-protein and fibre content makes them particularly good at regulating blood sugar levels, and therefore they are an excellent choice to prevent or treat hypoglycemia, diabetes, and insulin resistance; they also boost energy levels and help you lose weight. Extensive research on diets high in fibre like that found in chickpeas demonstrates their ability to reduce the risk of heart disease, heart attacks, and stroke. Their versatility makes them particularly popular in Indian curries, Middle Eastern dishes like hummus, and Mexican dishes. They can be added to soups, stews, and curries; puréed into a dip or sandwich spread; tossed onto a salad; or simply spiced and eaten. They make a delicious addition to many meals, and you'll enjoy them so much you'll probably forget how good they are for you.

Chili Peppers—Not only do chili peppers pack a powerful punch to just about any recipe, but they give the fat metabolism in your body a serious kick. Chili peppers are one of the best foods for fighting fat, plus they contain a potent substance called capsaicin that depletes a compound called substance P, which is linked to pain in your body. What could be better than a food that simultaneously burns fat and reduces pain? What's more, a single chili pepper also provides a significant amount of vitamin C and beta carotene. So, as you've probably already guessed, chili peppers have a rightful place in the life force diet. Keep in mind that pickled chili peppers are typically loaded with preservatives and are not a suitable alternative to the fresh ones.

Garlic—Ancient Egyptians held garlic as sacred and even placed clay versions of garlic bulbs in the tomb of Tutankhamen. In a less mystical sounding practice, ancient Roman soldiers used to place cloves of garlic between their toes before heading off to battle, to help ward off infection. More recently, the National Cancer Institute is investigating this herb for its impressive anti-cancer properties. Additionally, garlic is anti-bacterial, anti-viral, and anti-fungal. Over 1000 scientific studies demonstrate the value of garlic, particularly its chemical component, allicin.

Kidney Beans—Taking its name from its kidney shape, kidney beans are high in protein (a cup provides 15.3 grams or almost one-third of your daily requirement) fibre, and minerals like molybdenum, iron, magnesium, potassium, folate (vitamin B9), and vitamin B1. The fibre found in kidney beans helps bind to excess cholesterol and escort it out of the body. The folate found in kidney beans helps to lower levels of homocysteine in the body, a substance that in high levels is a risk factor for heart disease or stroke. With their added dose of the body's own calcium channel blocker—magnesium—kidney beans pack a potent double-dose of protection against heart disease. While their obvious use is in chili, kidney beans can also be added to soups, tacos, salads, and stew or puréed along with some spices into a delicious bean dip or sandwich spread.

Jerusalem Artichokes—Not related to the green globe artichokes most people are familiar with, these knobby, root-type vegetables are sometimes called sunchokes after their sunflower relatives. When cooked, they have a delicate flavour similar to potatoes, but unlike white potatoes, they gently release their carbohydrates to provide fuel for your body, without the blood sugar fluctuations. Their valuable fibre, called inulin, has even been found to be beneficial for balancing blood sugar levels, and may be helpful for people suffering from diabetes, Syndrome X, or Metabolic Syndrome. Inulin is also known as a "prebiotic" since it feeds healthy bacteria in the intestines. Inulin also binds with toxins in the intestines to assist with their removal from the body. As if all of that wasn't good enough, studies show that inulin helps lower cholesterol and is a good source of iron.

Navy Beans—Contrary to what the name would suggest, navy beans are actually white, not blue. They are called navy beans because they were a staple food of the American navy at the beginning of the 20th century. Loaded with protein, complex carbohydrates (the good kind), fibre, and folate (vitamin B9), navy beans are an excellent Life Force Silver Food. They help to regulate blood sugar levels, which in turn help with weight loss and cravings, and help keep you feeling full for hours. They are helpful in warding off diabetes and hypoglycemia, and lower cholesterol levels.

Peas—Packed with important nutrients like vitamins A, B1, B6, C, K, and folate, beta carotene, iron, potassium, magnesium, zinc, and fibre, peas are a great part of the life force diet. You can add them to soups, stews, or curries, or, if they are fresh, you can even snap them out of their pods and eat them uncooked (a Life Force Gold Food) as a delicious snack. I love going to the market and eating fresh peas directly from their pods. Their impressive combination of nutrients helps to make them superb bone builders, and their high levels of folate and B6 make them excellent homocysteine reducers, which you may recall is a substance that in high levels is a risk factor for heart disease or stroke. You can enjoy peas uncooked, steamed, sautéed, in curries, soups and in stews.

Pinto Beans—Like other legumes, pinto beans are high in protein, complex carbohydrates, and fibre. Actually, a cup of cooked pinto beans contains more than 25 percent of your daily protein requirements. Additionally, they are a good source of the minerals molybdenum, manganese, iron, magnesium, potassium, and vitamin B1. In a study of over 40,000 male health professionals over four years, researchers found that men who ate the highest amount of fibre along with diets high in magnesium and potassium had a substantially reduced risk of stroke.[11] While good for just about everyone, pinto beans are particularly helpful for menstruating women since they are a good source of energy-boosting, blood-building iron. And, unlike their red meat counterparts, the iron found in pinto beans is free of harmful saturated fats. A cup of cooked pinto beans can provide almost one-quarter of your body's daily requirements for iron and with 14 grams of protein, they also provide over 28 percent of your daily protein needs. Bean dip, anyone?

Pumpkin—Possibly one of the foods that helped early European settlers in North America survive their first winter months, pumpkin is an excellent source of complex carbohydrates that help provide essential energy to the body, fibre to keep the bowels moving properly, and beta carotene (as its orange colour indicates). Pumpkin is an excellent addition to your diet and can be roasted, baked, or mashed, and added to soups, stews, bread, curries, and, of course, pumpkin pie. Be aware that most canned or store-bought prepared pumpkin tends to be high in fat or sugar. Avoid pumpkin that contains either and opt instead for whole pumpkins or canned pumpkin without additives. It's easy to cook small pre-washed pumpkins in a small amount of water overnight on low in a slow cooker. Let cool and then scoop out the seeds and cut away the stem. Purée in the blender or food processor and add to recipes.

Quinoa—A nutty-tasting grain that was a staple in the diet of ancient Incas, who gave it the name "mother grain," quinoa is an excellent source of protein, fibre, numerous B-vitamins, and the minerals potassium, manganese, magnesium, iron, and zinc. Quinoa helps ward off heart disease, migraines, and heart arrhythmias. Because it cooks in 20 minutes or less, it is a great alternative to white rice. Plus, it is nutritionally superior to white rice in every way and tastes better too. There are two types: regular quinoa and the debittered variety. Both are excellent choices. Simply choose the one that you enjoy most. It can be used in recipes that call for rice or couscous. I also enjoy it with some almond milk and a small amount of pure maple syrup as a warming winter breakfast. Check the grain cooking chart on page 204 to learn how to cook this yummy grain.

Red Peppers—While all bell peppers are Life Force Silver Foods, red peppers are particularly packed in nutrients like vitamins A and C, making them an especially good addition to your diet. You can also eat them in an uncooked state, in which case they would be considered Life Force Gold Foods, due to their enzymes being intact. Red peppers also contain vitamin B6, vitamin B1, folate, and lycopene, a phytonutrient that has been linked to a reduced risk of cervical, pancreatic, and bladder cancers. The fibre found in red peppers binds to cancer-causing toxins in the intestines, escorting them out of your body.[12] An incredibly versatile food, red bell peppers can be added to soups, stews, salads, and wraps; roasted and added to sandwiches; puréed into dip; and served in many other ways.

Salmon (Wild)—An excellent source of inflammation-taming Omega 3s, wild salmon also provides superior protein to other animal sources of protein. Wild salmon contains many of the B-complex vitamins, vitamin D, and minerals such as calcium, potassium, and selenium. Because of its anti-inflammatory abilities, eating wild salmon one to three times weekly can help ward off heart disease, arthritis, Alzheimer's disease, stroke, and many other health concerns. You may recall our earlier discussion about the insufficient quantities of Omega 3 fatty acids in the typical North American diet. Wild salmon helps to counter the imbalance. Steam, pan-fry over low to medium heat, grill, or poach wild salmon to enjoy its delicious taste and many nutritious qualities.

Squash—Like its relative, the pumpkin, squash is an excellent source of complex carbohydrates, fibre, and beta carotene, making it a delicious and nutritious addition to your life force diet. Use it as you might use pumpkin, or roast wedges and serve on salad, in wraps, or on sandwiches.

Sweet Potatoes—High in beta carotene, C, and B6, as well as potassium, iron, and magnesium, sweet potatoes are naturally delicious and nutritionally superior to white potatoes. Their rich orange colour indicates that they are high in beta carotene, which is the precursor to vitamin A in your body. There are so many great ways to enjoy sweet potatoes in your diet. Try them roasted, puréed, steamed, baked, or grilled. You can add them to soups and stews, or grill and place on top of leafy greens for a delicious life force salad. I enjoy grilling them with onions and red peppers for amazing sandwich or wrap ingredients.

Tomatoes—Packed with vitamin C and an important phytonutrient called lycopene, tomatoes are an excellent addition to your diet. Lycopene has been studied extensively for its antioxidant effects against aging and disease and its anti-cancer properties. It even demonstrates the incredible ability to protect genetic material against disease and damage. Lycopene appears to be particularly effective against colon and prostate cancers. You can enjoy tomatoes cooked or uncooked. While you will obtain more vitamin C from uncooked tomatoes, lycopene is best absorbed from cooked tomatoes. I recommend eating both types on a regular basis to enjoy the best nutritional and taste benefits. You can add tomatoes to soups, stews, curries, salads, sandwiches, and salsas.

Wild Rice—Not a true grain, wild rice is actually a type of aquatic grass seed native to the United States and Canada. It tends to be a bit pricier than other grains, but its high content of protein and nutty flavour make wild rice worth every penny. It is an excellent choice for people with celiac disease or who have gluten or wheat sensitivities. Wild rice is an excellent food to boost energy levels since it is high in complex carbohydrates and helps keep blood sugar levels stable thanks to its fibre content. Add wild rice to soups, stews, salads, and pilaf. It is important to note that wild rice is black. There are many blends of white and wild rice, which are considerably higher in carbs and tend to consist primarily of refined white rice. Be sure to use only wild rice, not the blends that are mostly white rice with a handful of wild rice.

6

Week Three—Next, Go for the Gold!

*"The food we put in our systems determines the
health of every cell and organ in our bodies. The
human body needs live foods to build 'live cells.'"*

—Jay Kordich, "The Juiceman"

HIPPOCRATES, a Greek physician born almost 2500 years ago and
known as the "father of medicine," wrote: "Let food be thy medicine
and medicine be thy food." By week three, I bet that you are beginning to recognize the role of food as medicine. Not only can food
heal disease, but in many cases it can prevent illness altogether.

By now you are probably surprised at how easy it is to eat healing
foods like leafy greens, wild salmon, and wild rice and enjoy their
delicious taste. Most people are shocked by how wonderful the Life
Force Silver Foods actually are. Since your body has been given a
break from junk and processed foods, it has been able to improve
its detox mechanisms to start eliminating toxins from the fat stores
in your body. By eating nutrient-rich Life Force Silver Foods your
body's own enzyme processes have been enhanced to improve the
trillions of cellular functions that give you energy, manufacture and
balance hormones, and balance your weight. You have most likely

noticed a difference in how you feel. After week two most people have noticed a definite increase in energy, experience less heaviness and bloating, feel mentally alert, and have even experienced weight loss (if they were overweight).

If you haven't seen these types of health improvements, don't worry. It's important to remember that your body is working at the cellular level to restore health and vitality so that the results are long lasting and more effective than fad diets that offer quick and short-lived results. While your cells' trillions of functions may have improved, they simply may not have translated into symptom improvement yet. Everyone's body is different. It's important to trust the innate intelligence that coordinates the functions in your body. Some people experience rapid results while others take longer. The timing can depend on many factors, but certainly the level of toxins in your body and how healthy or ill you were prior to starting the life force diet play a role. Regardless of the improvements you've experienced, in week three, we'll be ramping up your enzyme functions even further by escalating the amount of enzymes you ingest through the amazing Life Force Gold Foods. Like their name indicates, these foods are nature's life force–enhancing powerhouses.

While we could have drastically altered your diet on the first day to eat nothing but Life Force Gold Foods, typically that approach is ineffective. Most people who attempt such drastic changes also experience drastic detoxification symptoms. While it's common to hear people referring to the headaches, fatigue, diarrhea, bloating, achiness, and many other negative symptoms as a "healing crisis," I disagree. These symptoms are the signs that your body's detoxification systems are overloaded and cannot handle the many toxins that are stirred up by making drastic dietary changes. So, by making these changes over three weeks, you're much less likely to experience any of these negative symptoms and are likely already to be experiencing greater energy and vitality. The life force diet, while designed for rapid health improvements over three weeks, offers you the tremendous rewards of vibrant health, youthful good looks, immunity against disease, and powerful vitality when continued for life.

This week you'll learn what foods fall into the Life Force Gold Food category, how much you should eat, when to eat them for the best results, and how easy it can be to add more of them to your diet. You will be asked to focus on organic foods (as you increase your consumption of uncooked foods to 50 percent, high-quality produce becomes vital). You will also be adding at least three servings per week of fermented foods, as well as one or two helpings of delicious, enzyme-powered sprouts.

I'm sure you have been eating salads and greens and maybe even some fruit shakes over the past two weeks. But this chapter is going to show you how to easily ramp that up until a full 50 percent of your diet is derived from enzyme-dense, Life Force Gold Foods. You will need to carefully read the information below to get a great under-standing of what makes each of these natural powerhouses so vital to this final week (and the rest of your eating days), and then spend the week ensuring that at every meal, at least half of your plate is made up of these outrageously delicious foods. It is only a week—and you can do it. Of course, I invite you to keep eating the life force way for all of your days, but please, make a commitment now to plan out this last week and really experience the difference that enzymes can make in every aspect of your health.

Once we have taken a look at each of these new dietary ad-ditions in detail, I will give you a comprehensive list of the most powerful Life Force Gold Foods, detailing their incredible vitamin, mineral, and enzyme content. You will be able to pick anything from this list to add to your already healthier diet. We will discuss ways to increase the amount of uncooked foods you eat (including adding avocado to stews, colourful vegetables to soups after they have been removed from the heat, and salsa to almost anything), and, finally, I will leave you with my top 14 tips for success. This chapter will give you everything you need to know about the most incredible healing foods on our planet, and how to incorporate them into your diet. And for those of you who would prefer not to have to experiment on your own in the kitchen, you can turn to Chapter 9 for a whole host of recipes to get you started.

What Are Life Force Gold Foods?

Simply put, Life Force Gold Foods are those that are packed with life force enzymes. As you now know, all foods contain enzymes in their natural state, but heating over 118 degrees Fahrenheit, canning, and processing destroys the enzymes they contain. Life Force Gold Foods are those that are natural, health-building foods that contain plentiful amounts of nutrients and enzymes and are eaten and/or prepared in a way in which the enzymes remain intact.

Does that mean you need to swear off all cooked foods in favour of an exclusively raw foods diet? No; of course not! There's nothing radical about the life force diet other than its miraculous ability to restore great health, energy, and immunity.

There's no need to worry about which Life Force Gold Foods are best. As I commonly tell people, "The best Life Force Foods are the ones you actually eat." Start eating those on the list that you know and love, and give your less-than-favourite ones another try. Sometimes it's as simple as a new way of preparing foods or combining them with different flavours to love foods you couldn't stand before.

Going for Gold

Let's take a look at a sampling of the Life Force Gold Foods. Don't worry if you're not familiar with them all. Neither was I when I first started eating this way! But, over time, I made wonderful food discoveries that I want to share with you. Feel free to copy this list and post it on your fridge for those moments when you feel at a loss as to what to eat—just look at all of these delicious foods!

Life Force Gold Foods

Beverages

Freshly-squeezed fruit and vegetable juices (diluted 1:1 with water)

Life Force Lemonade (recipe at the back of the book)

Fruits

Black currants	Mangoes
Blackberries	Nectarines
Blueberries	Oranges
Cantaloupe	Papaya
Cherries	Peaches
Clementines	Pears
Dates	Persimmons
Figs	Pineapple
Goji berries	Pomegranates
Gooseberries	Prunes (unsulphured/without
Grapefruit	sulphites)
Grapes (red or green)	Quince
Guava	Raisins (all varieties, unsulphured/
Honeydew melon	without sulphites)
Kiwi fruit	Raspberries
Kumquat	Red or green grapes
Lemons	Strawberries
Limes	Watermelon
Lychee	Watermelon
Mandarins and tangerines	Yellow or orange peppers

Herbs and Spices*

Basil	Ginger
Chilies	Horseradish
Chives	Marjoram
Cilantro	Mint

Continued on page 148

Continued from page 147

Life Force Gold Foods

Herbs and Spices*

Parsley	Any other fresh, uncooked
Rosemary	herbs and spices
Sage	Miscellaneous Cacao beans
Thyme	Cacao nibs
Turmeric root	Cacao paste

Nuts and Nut Butters***

Almonds	Macadamia nuts
Almond butter	Macadamia nut butter
Brazil nuts	Pecans
Brazil nut butter	Pecan butter
Cashews	Pinenuts (pignolia nuts)
Cashew butter	Pistachios
Hazelnuts	Walnuts
Hazelnut butter	Walnut butter

Oils**

Almond Oil	Hempseed Oil
Coconut Oil	Olive Oil
Flaxseed Oil/Flax Oil	Sesame Oil
Grapeseed Oil	Sunflower Oil
Hazelnut Oil	Walnut Oil

Seeds and Seed Butters***

Chia seeds	Pumpkin seed butter
Flaxseeds	Sesame seeds
Hemp seeds	Sunflower seeds
Hemp butter	Sunflower butter
Pumpkin seeds	Tahini (raw)

Sprouts

Aduki bean sprouts	Amaranth sprouts
Alfafa sprouts	Broccoli sprouts

Buckwheat sprouts	Mustard sprouts
Cabbage sprouts	Oat sprouts
Clover sprouts	Onion sprouts
Fenugreek sprouts	Pinto bean sprouts
Garbanzo bean	Quinoa sprouts
(chickpea) sprouts	Radish sprouts
Garlic sprouts	Rye sprouts
Kale sprouts	Spelt sprouts
Kamut sprouts	Sunflower sprouts
Lentil sprouts	

Vegetables

Beet greens	Mushrooms
Beetroot	Onions
Cabbage (purple, green,	Radishes
or Chinese)	Red (or yellow or
Carrots	orange) peppers
Celery	Sea vegetables (such as agar,
Cucumbers	arame, dulse, kelp, wakame, etc.)
Daikon	Shallots
Green beans	Sorrel
Green peppers	Spinach
Hot peppers	Tomatoes
Leafy green vegetables	Watercress
Leeks	Yacon chips (raw)
Lettuce	Yacon root
Mâche	Yellow or orange peppers

* Fresh, uncooked herbs and spices only

**All oils should be eaten in modest amounts only. Use cold-pressed or extra virgin oils. Flax oil should be refrigerated.

*** Raw, unpasteurized nuts and nut butters only. Ideally, soak nuts and seeds overnight and drain before eating.

You many notice some of the same foods on both the list of Life Force Silver Foods and Life Force Gold Foods. These foods have excellent medicinal properties when eaten either cooked or uncooked. Only uncooked foods contain potent healing enzymes—enzymes are what make Gold Foods gold—but both Gold and Silver Foods have plentiful amounts of vitamins and minerals.

Ignite Your Life Force

> **STEP 18 Go for the Gold!**
>
> This week make sure that Life Force Gold Foods make up at least 50 percent of everything you eat. Life Force Gold Foods are uncooked fruits, vegetables, sea vegetables, sprouts, sprouted grains, and sprouted legumes. It's easy to do by drinking a fresh juice or two, eating a large green salad with meals, snacking on fruit or raw nuts, adding a large handful of sprouts to sandwiches, or tossing bean sprouts on your cooked stir-fries.

Revitalize Your Body with Enzymes

By now you've likely noticed that your cravings for unhealthy foods are subsiding, your body is moving toward greater health, and the introduction of a diet that is 50 percent uncooked, enzyme-rich foods will give your body a total health revolution. You've probably noticed that your tiredness has disappeared, your skin is clearer, your thinking is incredibly clearer and more focused, and any excess weight you've been carrying is on the way out.

According to many experts, the more enzyme-depleted foods we eat, the faster we exhaust our internal supplies, and the result is exhaustion, weight gain, accelerated aging, and the onset of illness. But there's good news! By eating a diet high in enzyme-rich life force foods, we can often reverse these problems, as well as turn back the clock on aging! Life force foods are the key to weight loss, mental clarity, boundless energy, and radiant good looks. And if you have any doubts, try *The Life Force Diet*. As the old adage states, "The proof is in the pudding." In this case, you'll be amazed at all the health benefits you'll experience by following an enzyme-rich diet. What's more, there are absolutely no harmful side effects from following this diet.

I will describe exactly which foods will help your body return to its healthiest, most attractive state. It's really quite simple: 50 percent of all foods are eaten in their natural, unadulterated state, with all the enzymes left intact. We call these Life Force Gold Foods, including blueberries, cherries, avocados, leafy greens, bean sprouts, almonds, pecans, bananas, raspberries, coconut, and many others. The remaining 50 percent of life force foods include Life Force Silver Foods: wild and brown rice, fish, beans, vegetables, and whole grains. If you're eating animal protein then 35 percent of life force foods include Life Force Silver Foods and up to 15 percent will be comprise organic meat, poultry, fish, and eggs. The beauty of this superior eating plan is that it satisfies the cravings created by empty-calorie foods by replacing them with delicious!—even decadent!—foods. And you'll never feel better!

It's easy to get 50 percent of your diet in the form of Life Force Gold Foods. Let's explore breakfast options first.

Life Force Breakfast Ideas

We've all heard the adage that breakfast is the most important meal of the day: It's no different on the life force diet. Start with a piece or two of fruit, or a small bowl of berries. They're best eaten on an empty stomach, particularly in the morning. If possible, eat the rest of your breakfast about half an hour later. This break helps the fruit to be digested quickly and unimpeded by other foods. Then you can choose from any number of options, depending on your personal preferences. You can have organic eggs with a piece of sprouted grain bread, a fruit and almond milk smoothie, a veggie-tofu scrambler, a pudding made from blending half an avocado with your favourite fruit such as Strawberry-Blueberry Pudding on page 255, or a Japanese-style breakfast such as Miso Soup on page 236.

Life Force Lunch and Dinner

The possibilities for lunches and dinners are endless. You can enjoy delicious pastas or noodle dishes by choosing brown rice or spelt pasta and topping it with a fresh tomato sauce, Life Force Salsa, or Alfredo Sauce (see Pasta Alfredo with Asparagus on page 251). Add a large green salad and a fresh carrot or veggie juice and you have the perfect ratios of Life Force Gold and Silver Foods. If you're looking for a light lunch, choose Roasted Carrot Soup and a salad, or simply go with a large Life Force Salad, which is a delicious meal on its own. Enjoy a lentil burger on a whole grain spelt bun or cut into slices, topped with greens, tomato, and sprouts and added to a sprouted grain wrap. Or have a small serving of grilled wild salmon and a Salade du Provence for an amazing dinner. On a cold winter evening you might prefer Savoury Lentil Stew with Life Force Tortilla Chips.

Fruit—Detox Powerhouses

I'm always astounded when clients arrive in my office telling me that they don't eat fruit. When I ask them, "Why not?" they inform me that they are too high in carbs and cause weight gain. Almost always, when I investigate to learn more about their diet, I find that these people eat chocolate bars or other sweets, or regularly drink "diet" cola or some other sugary beverage.

While fruit does contain carbs, remember: Your body needs healthy carbs as an energy source. Fruit is among nature's finest foods to assist with cleansing your body. Additionally, most fruit contains high amounts of vitamins, minerals, and enzymes if eaten in its natural, raw state. Like their vegetable counterparts, most fruit is high in important phytonutrients that help our bodies prevent or fight disease, or burn fat. Follow the suggestions below for consuming fruit. If you're trying to lose weight, it's best to limit your fruit consumption to two to three servings a day.

Typically, the deeper and darker the colour of the fruit, the higher it is in important phytonutrients. You may remember our discussion on anthocyanins in the last chapter. Fruits are also packed with many macronutrients, vitamins, minerals, and other phytonutrients as well as fibre—all of which are critical to great health as you learned earlier. If you're not eating fruit, I highly recommend that you start doing so. If you're among the people who claim they cannot handle fruit, you may want to revisit our discussion on digestion on page 55 or address a possible intestinal candida overgrowth.

Additionally, because fruits are quickly digested, it is advisable to follow the following simple suggestions when eating them.

Ignite Your Life Force

STEP 19 Optimize Your Life Force Gold Fruit Digestion

1. Eat fruit on an empty stomach at least half an hour before meals or one hour after meals (longer if the meal was heavy). I usually eat fruit first thing in the morning, get ready for my day, and then eat other foods for breakfast.

2. It is fine to use small amounts of fruit on green salads or as part of a salad dressing. It's fine to mix fruit and vegetables if you're ingesting them in the form of juices because with the fibre removed they are both readily absorbed. Whenever you're drinking juices—fruit or vegetable or a combination of both— it's best to dilute them with equal parts of water to juice. One of my favourite juice combinations is carrot, apple, and ginger. I also love lemon, carrot, and apple juice. When I make green juices full of green veggies, I often add an apple to sweeten them slightly and make them more palatable.

3. Chew fruit well. Fruit's healthy and complete digestion depends partly on being chewed well, since chewing helps to break

down the fibre, release the fruit's own enzymes, and mix it with the body's digestive juices. When all of these things happen, fruit will be almost completely digested in the upper chamber of the stomach within the first half hour of eating it.

4. Use moderation when consuming fruit. Choose fruit over other types of sweets, but if you have a tendency to overeat sweets, do not replace one addiction with another.

Sprouts—Life Force Superstars

Sprouts offer an extraordinary amount of life force and a remarkable amount of nutrients. During the sprouting process, when seeds, nuts, grains, or beans are soaked in water and then sprouted, a tremendous amount of life force is ignited and nutrients that were locked inside are released and multiplied. At the same time the protein, complex carbohydrates (the good kind), and fatty acids also increase in quantity and value. This is because the enzymes in the seed become active and initiate digestion of these macronutrients, making it easier to digest and assimilate their nutrients when you eat them.

Sprouts are packed with healing enzymes that can dramatically improve health. It is not essential to eat sprouts on the life force diet if you simply can't stand them. However, I encourage you to try them since they offer the greatest life force and healing power of any foods. Whether you are suffering from severe fatigue, digestive troubles, depression, or cancer, sprouts' powerhouse of enzyme and nutrients can help.

Experts estimate that there can be up to 100 times more enzymes in sprouts than in uncooked fruits and vegetables, depending on the particular enzyme and seed sprouted. Typically, the greatest period of enzyme activity in sprouts is between germination and one week.[1] The type of sprout will determine which enzymes are present. In nature's wisdom, a particular sprout will include all the enzymes required to digest it, thereby ensuring improved digestion and assimilation of nutrients.

Research shows that some impressive changes take place in seeds that are sprouted, making them a great source of nutrition. Following are a few of these changes:

1. **The quality of protein in the seeds, grain, or beans improves.** The proteins in grains change form during soaking or sprouting, which improves the nutritional value. One particular amino acid called lysine, which is needed to prevent cold sores and to maintain a healthy immune system, increases during this process.[2]

2. **Fibre content of the seeds, grains, or beans increases.** In one study, fibre content in barley seeds increased from 3.75 percent of the seed to 6 percent of the sprout[3]—a significant increase. Since most of us are not getting adequate fibre, adding sprouts to our foods can be an excellent way to increase this valuable nutrient.

3. **Essential fatty acids increase during the sprouting process.**[4] These are the healthy fats our bodies need and few of us get adequate amounts in our diet.

4. **Vitamin content increases, particularly vitamins A, B-complex, C, and E.** The vitamin content of some seeds, grains, or beans can increase up to 20 times their original value within a few days of sprouting. Mung bean sprouts are an excellent example. You are probably already familiar with these sprouts, which are usually just called "bean sprouts" and are frequently used in many Asian dishes. Research shows that the sprouting process increases vitamins B1 up to 285 percent, B2 up to 515 percent, and niacin up to 256 percent.[5]

During the sprouting process, minerals found in the seed, grain, or bean bind to protein, making them more usable in the body.[6] Normally, this is a process that occurs within the body during digestion.

Ignite Your Life Force

> **STEP 20** **Step Up Your Life Force with Enzyme-Packed Sprouts**
>
> If you've never given sprouts a try, now is the time to do so. They are so easy to add to your diet. Here are some ways to help you get started:
>
> - Add a handful to your favourite salad recipe.
> - Throw a large handful of mung bean sprouts into your favourite noodle dish or stir-fry after you've removed it from the heat and are ready to serve it.
> - Add alfalfa or clover sprouts to a sandwich or wrap.
> - If you want to spice up a salad or sandwich, add some mustard, radish, or fenugreek sprouts for instant flavour.
> - Mung bean sprouts make a delicious salad alongside your favourite veggies. Simply add grated or julienned (cut into matchsticks) vegetables like red or green peppers, carrots, celery, cucumbers or any others you prefer. Toss in a dressing such as the Life Force Salad Dressing or the Thai Noodle Salad Dressing (see recipes in Chapter 9).

FAQ: I read articles in my newspaper stating that alfalfa and bean sprouts cause food poisoning. Is that true?

Answer: Like almost every other food, sprouts can be vulnerable to salmonella. Any food, utensil, or work surface can become contaminated with salmonella bacteria, which can lead to food poisoning in humans. The most common culprits are raw and undercooked meat, especially chicken and eggs, fish, peanut butter, sauces, and salad dressings. There are no visible signs, nor is there necessarily an odour that emanates from the contaminated food.

In healthy people, food poisoning, or salmonellosis as it is also called, can cause flu-like symptoms, including extreme headache, stomach cramps, vomiting, fever, nausea, and diarrhea. But sprouts are no more prone to salmonella bacteria than any other food, and they offer substantially more health benefits than risk.

Here's how you can minimize your risk of food poisoning with any foods:

1. Always wash your hands thoroughly (at least 20 seconds with natural soap and water) prior to handling or preparing food.
2. Always use clean utensils.
3. Sanitize your cutting board regularly between uses. Two great natural options are white vinegar or hydrogen peroxide (3 percent). If you're using the latter, be sure to set the board on paper towels away from any surfaces or fabrics that might be susceptible to bleaching, since hydrogen peroxide can have a bleaching effect. Both vinegar and hydrogen peroxide are effective against salmonella and other bacteria. I keep a spray bottle of them under the sink for easy and regular use.
4. Always wash sprouts you purchase or grow at home just prior to using.
5. When cooking meat, fish, or poultry, always be sure the temperature is hot enough to kill any bacteria—the temperature at the core of the meat should be at least 145 to 185 degrees Fahrenheit (63 to 85 degrees Celsius). Poultry should always be on the highest side of this range. And remember if you choose to eat animal products like meat, eggs, fish, or poultry, choose only organic meat, eggs, and poultry, and wild-caught fish. Keep their consumption to 15 percent of your daily diet.

The Case for Organic Foods

In the third week of the life force diet you are providing your body with the highest quality and most nutrient-rich food to help it restore you to great and vibrant health. Organic food is food in the state that nature intended it and provides higher nutritional value than conventional produce. Consuming organic produce as much as possible on the life force diet frees your body from attempting to detoxify pesticide residues or trying to deal with much of our food supply's genetically modified DNA. Let's explore the case for organic foods.

There have been two main arguments against buying and eating organic food. First, critics state that the nutritional difference between organic and conventional (using chemical herbicides, pesticides and/or fertilizers) fruits and vegetables is negligible. The second argument is that organic produce costs too much. There is no shortage of evidence demonstrating the value of organic foods from a health and nutritional perspective. I would also debate whether the cost argument holds much weight these days. Besides, you'll be eliminating the costlier processed, prepared, and packaged foods, as well as reducing or eliminating meat, all of which substantially increase the final price of your grocery bill.

The majority of research on organic food is conducted overseas in Europe, Australia, and Asia. In North America, many decades of investment in industrial agriculture methods have all but eliminated organic farming from the map. Fortunately, it is making a comeback and prompting renewed interest in research. Australia and Asian and European countries have remained more open to accepting organic farming and are equally receptive to funding research on how food, pesticides, herbicides, and genetic modification may affect human health.

Virginia Worthington, Doctor of Science and a certified nutrition specialist at Johns Hopkins University's School of Public Health, reviewed 41 published studies comparing the nutritional value of organically grown and conventionally grown fruits, vegetables, and grains. She concluded that there are significantly more of several nutrients in organic crops—27 percent more vitamin C, 21.1 percent more iron, 29.3 percent more magnesium, and 13.6 percent more phosphorus. The research also indicated that organic products had 15.1 percent fewer nitrates than their conventional counterparts. Worthington also compared five servings of organic vegetables (lettuce, spinach, carrots, potatoes, and cabbage) to the equivalent serving of conventionally grown vegetables. She found that only the organic servings provided the recommended daily intake of vitamin C for men and women. Worthington said the results are consistent with known soil dynamics and plant physiology.[7]

Research from Newcastle University in the United Kingdom reported that organically produced food had higher levels of specific antioxidants and lower mycotoxin (a fungal infection that can affect food crops) levels than conventional samples. The same research found that grass-based organic cattle diets reduce the risk of *E. coli* contamination while grain-based conventional diets increase the risk.

An Italian study conducted by the Istituto nazionale di ricerca per gli alimenti e la nutrizione (National Institute of Food and Nutrition Research) reported that organic pears, peaches, and oranges had higher antioxidant levels than their conventional counterparts. This multi-year study found that organic pears contained less fibre than those grown conventionally; however, they had more natural sugar, vitamin C, and other antioxidants. Interestingly, they were more resistant to mildew and fungi— an argument often used against organic food production, which is mistakenly viewed as more susceptible to pests. While the researchers did not report phytonutrient content, mildew and fungi resistance may also indicate higher phytonutrient content in the organic crops. I'd be curious to see this tested as well.[8]

The second argument regarding cost will continue to lose steam as organic food returns to popularity and greater availability; however, almost everyone will find that by removing the 3 Ps from your shopping list and replacing them with organic whole foods, your weekly shopping order will *decrease* in cost. The same is true of organic meat and eggs. While they tend to cost a bit more, you'll be eating less of them, if you're eating them at all.

Ignite Your Life Force

STEP 21 Choose Organic as Much as Possible

By giving your body pure organic food devoid of harmful pesticides (that your body must use its precious energy to detoxify) and genetically modified DNA, you lessen the burden on your body's energy reserves. In the case of non-organic meat and eggs, your body will have to detoxify the antibiotics, growth and other hormones, and other drugs and substances given to animals. Organic meat and eggs are free of these harmful substances. Organic food typically has higher nutritional value and just tastes better. Your body deserves the best quality food to build the best quality cells. Choose organic produce and meat as much as possible.

Fermented Foods

I mentioned earlier that fermented soy foods like miso and tempeh are easiest for the body to digest and absorb. Other naturally fermented foods are valuable additions to your diet. They are typically easier to digest and therefore their ingredients are better assimilated. They also offer valuable probiotics—the beneficial bacteria needed for a healthy body. In addition to the many fermented soy foods I mentioned earlier, you may also wish to add pickled ginger and sauerkraut. Keep in mind that I am referring to unsweetened, preservative- and artificial colour-free choices that are best found in a natural foods store.

Ignite Your Life Force

> **STEP 22** **Don't Forget the Fermented Foods**
>
> Strive to include naturally fermented foods in your diet at least a few times a week. They include miso, sauerkraut, tempeh, or some of the other foods mentioned on page 126. The easiest way to do this is to enjoy a fermented food every other day. Don't worry if these foods are new to you. Many are incredibly delicious. Although I was unfamiliar with miso for most of my life, miso soup is one of my favourite comfort foods now. If you're finding this step hard to do, be sure you're supplementing with a broad spectrum probiotic (you'll learn more in the next chapter).

Boost Your Life Force Now!

Boosting your life force energy doesn't have to feel like work. Just by learning a few simple tricks you can have a great impact on your life force for the rest of your life. Plus, you'll be surprised how enjoyable they are.

. Start the day out with the juice of one lemon squeezed into pure water. Not only do lemons contain over 20 anti-cancer compounds, they help to quickly restore your body's pH. And you may recall that enzymes can only work under certain conditions, including a balanced body chemistry. While lemons are acidic, when the juice of freshly squeezed lemon juice in water is metabolized, it alkalizes your body to help reduce pain or headaches, improve your energy levels, and optimize your body's natural enzyme processes.

Eat fresh fruit in the morning. Fresh fruit is packed with vitamins, minerals, phytonutrients, and of course, enzymes. When eaten on an empty stomach the fruit passes through your digestive system quickly to provide you with a quick boost of energy (it also takes minimal energy to digest fruit) and a potent boost of enzymes.

Snack on fresh fruit between meals. By making fresh fruit like apples, bananas, papaya, kiwi, or other enzyme-packed fruit a snack, you'll help to maintain your energy levels, balance your blood sugar, and give your body a burst of healing enzymes.

Snack on raw, soaked nuts and seeds throughout the day. By soaking raw nuts for at least an hour (but preferably overnight) and then draining them, you help to quash enzyme inhibitors found in nuts while increasing the nutrient content of the nuts. Soaking them increases their water content and digestibility, helping to make sure your body can assimilate their rich calcium, magnesium, zinc, and Omega 3 fatty acid stores. Nuts also make a great snack because they help to keep blood sugar levels stable and that means weight loss, greater energy, and balanced moods for you.

Keep a tray of crudités (raw veggie sticks) to add to meals or snack on or add to your meals. You'll be far more likely to eat them on a regular basis if they are already cleaned, cut, and ready to go.

Eat a large raw salad at a minimum of one meal a day. That doesn't include iceberg lettuce topped with a starchy tomato. I'm talking about a large green salad, either Romaine, mesclun mix, or your favourite greens—just be sure they are actually green. But your salad doesn't have to be a boring plate of greens. Top with some fresh berries, garlic and ginger crisps (as in the Life Force Salad recipe on page 244), brown rice noodles, salsa, roasted vegetables, or raw walnuts. I've observed many converts from salad haters to salad lovers with a little creativity and some delicious recipes (the latter you'll find in Chapter 9).

Sip fresh juice. Drink water with fresh lemon or lime juice in the morning or throughout the day. Enjoy a smoothie made with fresh fruit and almond milk. Drink a freshly made veggie and/or carrot juice between meals. It's easier and more delicious than you think to drink fresh juices. Once you get in the habit of having fresh juice, you'll never want packaged or concentrated juices again. The added energy they'll give you over time will be reward for the minimal effort required to make them.

Make a salad smoothie. Sounds disgusting but you'll be surprised how delicious, filling, and nutritious this power drink can be. Toss a large handful of mild greens like Boston lettuce, Romaine lettuce, or spinach along with berries, frozen banana, almond milk, or other smoothie ingredients and blend for an instant "green drink." I opt for a salad smoothie when I'm pressed for time or am just feeling a little lazy and want my salad in a hurry.

Chew, chew, chew! We've discussed the importance of thoroughly chewing your food extensively but it cannot be overstated. If you do not chew your food properly, you miss a whole stage of digestion. If you have trouble chewing or wear dentures, opt for more smoothies, juices, soups, and puréed vegetables while cutting the remainder of your food into smaller, manageable pieces.

Add sprouts to salads, wraps, sandwiches, noodles, or stir-fries after they've finished cooking. Sprouts are diverse and versatile. If you don't like one kind, try another. See the "Ignite Your Life Force" box "Step Up Your Life Force with Enzyme-Packed Sprouts" for more ideas.

Add raw to everything! After you've cooked soups, stews, or other foods, remove from the heat and add a handful of soft raw foods like diced tomatoes, zucchini, or fresh herbs. Or top with some crunch by adding bean sprouts or chopped raw nuts to a noodle dish or soup.

Curb a sweet tooth with fruit (eaten at least one hour after you've finished your meal or on an empty stomach) or a delicious Life Force Gold dessert. If you opt for a dessert, reserve them for only a day or two per week. Eating dessert after every dinner and snacking on high-sugar sweets throughout the day is a bad habit that needs to be broken. That doesn't mean you can't eat delicious and nutritious life force desserts on occasion, but keep them as treats, not necessities. Eat fruit instead. Once you kick the regular dessert habit, you'll find that your taste buds change. Over time, you will need fewer sweets and ones with fewer sugars to feel satisfied. If you're still struggling with cravings, you may want to snack on more nuts or high-fibre foods throughout the day to keep your blood sugar levels stable, or add a chromium supplement along with your meals.

Take a high-potency digestive enzyme with meals. The enzymes found in Life Force Gold Foods can only digest the food itself, not the cooked foods in your meals. So add a digestive enzyme with meals to offset the need for your body's own digestive enzymes (and energy!). You'll learn more about digestive enzyme supplements in the next chapter.

Eat only until you are full. For many people eating has become a pastime rather than something to nourish their appetites and bodies. Reducing the amount you eat may increase longevity. Research shows that even slightly restricting caloric intake increases the lifespan of laboratory animals so this benefit may transfer to humans as well. That doesn't mean you should starve yourself, go hungry, or use this advice as an excuse to support an eating disorder. Eat until you feel full but not heavy. It may take some time to adjust to this concept. Most people eat until they are bloated and heavy feeling and mistake that as feeling "full." Stop well before that. Snack later if you become hungry again, but pay attention to your body's signals, not just to your eyes and taste buds.

Quick and Simple Ways to Increase the Life Force in Your Meals

It's easy to boost the life force enzyme content of any meal with a few simple tricks:

1. Add a handful of chopped fresh herbs to soups, salads, stew, or other dishes.
2. Add a scoop of fresh avocado to soups, salads, stew, or other dishes upon serving.

3. Throw a fresh, raw salsa on top of your favourite soup, stew, or salad. For cooked dishes, add the salsa when serving.
4. Snack on vegetable crudités with raw almond butter, hummus, guacamole, or salsa.
5. Snack on raw, soaked nuts throughout the day for life force energy, stabilized blood sugar, and loads of calcium.

Summary of the Life Force Diet—Week 3

1. Go for the Gold by eating 50 percent of your diet in its natural, uncooked form.
2. Start your day with a glass of pure water and fresh lemon juice.
3. Optimize your Life Force Gold fruit digestion by chewing well, eating it in moderation, preferably on an empty stomach.
4. Step up your life force with enzyme-packed sprouts such as bean sprouts, alfalfa sprouts, onion sprouts, or another type.
5. Choose organic foods as much as possible.
6. Don't forget to eat naturally fermented foods like miso, tempeh, or sauerkraut every other day.

Life Force Gold Foods

Start adding the following foods to your daily diet to obtain a minimum of 50 percent uncooked Life Force Gold Foods. Of course, you can always eat a higher percentage than that, but at least strive for 50 percent daily. It is not necessary to eat all of these foods every day. Instead, select a variety of different options of varying colours on a daily basis. And, if you absolutely detest a particular food, don't eat it. The life force diet is made to be flexible. You can easily choose other foods you might enjoy more. Give some new ones a try periodically though. Enjoy!

Alfalfa Sprouts—Like most sprouts, alfalfa sprouts are jam-packed with nutrients and enzymes, making them tops on the Life Force Gold list. During the sprouting process both the nutrient levels and the enzyme contents of foods skyrocket and, thanks to the latter, sprouts are easily digestible. While a biologist named Frank Bouer more recently discovered that alfalfa leaves contain eight important enzymes, the alfalfa plant has been used by natural medicine practitioners for hundreds, if not thousands of years, particularly to treat arthritis and other pain disorders, and to strengthen the blood and heart. Research shows that alfalfa is effective in combating high cholesterol levels and may be beneficial in preventing coronary artery disease and stroke. While I haven't seen any research on alfalfa's effects on hair loss, when eaten regularly this little marvel is reputed to stimulate hair growth. It is also a good source of vitamin K, which helps the body to use calcium and improve blood clotting. I add a handful of alfafa sprouts to sandwiches, wraps, and salads on a regular basis to benefit from their many health-giving qualities.

Almonds—As delicious as they are nutritious, raw, unsalted almonds are packed with magnesium, calcium, protein, and fibre. They are also a good source of B-complex vitamins, vitamin E, iron, and magnesium. Eaten as a snack throughout the day, they help to stabilize blood sugar levels, encourage fat loss in overweight individuals, increase energy, and balance moods. They are the perfect anti-stress food when eaten on a regular basis. Their fibre content binds to toxins in your body to help you detox. However, if you are susceptible to cold sores, you may want to moderate your almond intake, since their high levels of the amino acid arginine can trigger or worsen outbreaks. Keep in mind that it can be difficult to find truly unheated almonds even if they appear to be raw.

Apples—We've all heard the adage, "an apple a day keeps the doctor away," and provided that apple is an organic one, the saying holds some truth. Apples contain important vitamins, minerals, and enzymes. They also contain plentiful amounts of pectin, an important type of fibre that binds to heavy metals and other toxins in your body to help eliminate them from your body. Additionally, they contain an important phytonutrient called malic acid, which when ingested helps improve energy production in your body.

Apricots—A couple of years ago I lived in a quaint town in British Columbia called Lillooet, where apricot trees seemed to grow wild. Before most people were aware the fruit had ripened, the neighbouring black bears would come to town and shake the trees until the ground turned orange. Fortunately, that was usually all the bears wanted and then they'd head back to the forests they called home. Their wild instincts led them to these beta carotene–rich foods that help build natural immunity against infection and strengthen eyesight, for humans as well. Additionally, they contain a healthy dose of potassium, boron, and iron. I wasn't a huge fan of these little fruits, but after eating them fresh I was hooked. Eaten uncooked, these Life Force Gold Foods make a delicious snack, or pitted, make an excellent topping for salads.

Bananas—Thanks to the low-carb craze, bananas have gotten a bad reputation. I've even had clients swear off them only to devour chocolate bars laden with sugar, preservatives, and artificial flavours. Not a good idea. Bananas are nature's fast food: they're pre-packed and ready to eat at a moment's notice. Ripe bananas are highly digestible due to their rich enzyme content, which works to break down the fruit's starches into healthy sugars that provide fuel for your brain and body. Some of the sugars in bananas are called fructooligosaccharides, or FOS for short. FOS helps feed the healthy bacteria in your gut to improve digestion, brain health, your immune system, and much more. The specific type of fibre in bananas is called pectin and it not only binds to heavy metals in your body to help eliminate them, it also helps soothe heartburn, digestive tract inflammation, and even ulcers. As if that weren't enough, bananas are a good source of vitamin B6, potassium, and tryptophan. The latter is a precursor to the hormone serotonin, which is your body's natural anti-depressant, mood lifter, and sleep enhancer. Because bananas are frequently harvested in rainforests of South and Central Americas, choose fair trade organic ones that are devoid of ripening gases.

Bean Sprouts—Also called mung bean sprouts, these sprouts are loaded with easily digestible protein thanks to their plentiful stores of enzymes. Plus, they contain high amounts of vitamin C to help ward off infection, cancer, and heart disease. They are commonly found in Asian cuisines alongside noodle dishes, but are versatile enough to enjoy in many other ways. To keep them as a Life Force Gold Food replete with enzymes, I throw them into a noodle dish after the noodles have been cooked and removed from the heat. Adding them to a wrap or sandwich is also an excellent way to keep their enzymes intact.

Blueberries—Packed with nutrients like vitamins C, E, B2, niacin, folate, and minerals like iron, magnesium, manganese, and potassium, blueberries would be an incredible Life Force Food if that were all they offered. But they are loaded with phytonutrients as well, making this fruit a must-have in your daily diet. Some of their phytonutrients include anthocyanins, ellagic acid, quercetin, catechins, and salicylic acid. If the latter sounds familiar, you may recognize it as the drug we've come to know as Aspirin. That's right—blueberries contain natural aspirin, but in this beautiful and delicious packaging offered by Mother Nature, there's no worry about harmful side effects. What's more, blueberries are proven to reduce heat shock proteins that are linked with some forms of brain disease, making these little marvels potent weapons in the prevention of Alzheimer's and Parkinson's disease as well as other neurological disorders. You can reap their many body-balancing and disease-prevention benefits by adding them to your diet in the form of either fresh or frozen berries. I enjoy a regular bowl of frozen blueberries, thawed just slightly so they taste just like blueberry ice cream. Sometimes I'll purée them in a food processor with a frozen banana and a little water for a delicious blueberry-banana ice cream. But you can just as easily throw them in a smoothie for a breakfast-on-the-go or an afternoon pick-me-up.

Cantaloupe—As this melon's orange flesh would indicate, they are high in beta carotene, which helps strengthen your immune system against viruses and bacteria, while maintaining healthy eyesight. In studies, beta carotene has been shown to ward off the formation of cataracts. Cantaloupes also contain a good amount of vitamin C, potassium, and fibre. Beta carotene and vitamin C are both anti-oxidants that protect your body against free radicals linked to aging and disease. I enjoy eating fresh, uncooked cantaloupe on its own or as a component of a delicious fruit salad instead of less-than-healthy sweets. I also frequently top green salads with some thin slices of this fruit along with a citrus-based dressing for a delicious and super-healthy meal.

Cherries—I long for cherry season every year. I grew up in Hamilton, Ontario, which is along central Canada's fruit belt. Once I was old enough to drive, I would regularly head out along the escarpment to find the market stands displaying the growers' finest fruit and vegetable delights. Cherries were my first pick as soon as they were in season. I'd devour them by the handfuls and was always disappointed when cherry season was over. One of my favourite fruits, cherries are well-deserving of their place on the Life Force Gold Food list. Their rich reddish-purplish colour indicates their plentiful amounts of phytonutrients, particularly anthocyanins and quercetin, both of which have potent antioxidant properties. Remember that anthocyanins are powerful protectors against brain disease and quercetin helps alleviate breathing disorders, allergic reactions, and joint inflammation. Cherries are also an excellent source of numerous vitamins, including carotene and minerals like iron. Eat them fresh and uncooked to enjoy their plentiful nutrients and phytonutrients, while knowing that you're giving your body powerful medicine against disease—and cherries are better tasting than any pharmaceutical drugs!

Coconut—In India, the coconut is considered *kalpavriksha*, or "tree of life," making it a fitting addition to the life force diet. While this healthy food has gotten a bad reputation due to its saturated fat content, its saturated fats are in the form of "medium chain triglycerides," which, unlike saturated fats found in meat and dairy products, are good for your body and easy to digest. These excellent fats actually appear to increase energy production and fat burning! One type of fat found in coconut called lauric acid even converts to an antiviral and antibacterial substance in the body, thereby helping to increase immunity to viruses and bacteria. What's more, coconuts even contain an antifungal ingredient called caprylic acid. Raw coconut flesh can be eaten on its own, in dessert recipes, or as a salad topping. I melt raw coconut oil over extremely low heat and add to flax oil for a delicious and healthy butter substitute (see Michelle's Better Butter recipe on page 230). You can also use raw coconut oil on low to medium heat for cooking or in baked-good recipes. Coconut milk or coconut water can be added to soups, stews, curries, desserts, and much more.

Cranberries—Originally used by the First Nations of North America for urinary tract infections, cranberries and cranberry juice (the real deal, not the sugar-laden stuff most grocery stores dispense) are excellent Life Force Gold Foods, when eaten in their uncooked state. (Many unsweetened cranberry juices are pasteurized, making them Life Force Silver Foods). Either way, these tart fruits offer sweet healing against infections. According to researchers at the

Alliance City Hospital in Ohio, cranberries contain compounds that prevent *E. coli* bacteria from sticking to the walls of the urinary tract making it easier to be flushed out of the body. Cranberries and pure cranberry juice also appear to flush fat, toxins, and debris from the body's lymphatic system—a network of vessels and fluid that operates like an internal street-sweeper. In addition to their anti-bacterial properties, cranberries also have antiviral and antifungal properties, thereby helping your whole body to fight off infection. Plus, they're high in nutrients like vitamin C and potassium, and contain some folate and calcium. I throw a couple of handfuls of cranberries into a juicer or blender along with sweeter fruit like apples, bananas, or blueberries for a delicious smoothie.

Cucumbers—Cucumbers have been used traditionally for their skin-healing properties but have many other benefits as well. The skins of cucumbers contain plant sterols, which are basically plant hormones. In our bodies these sterols reduce elevated cholesterol levels, making cucumbers helpful against heart disease. High in both water and minerals, cucumbers help to lower blood pressure, flush toxins out of the kidneys, and work as an excellent bodily detoxifier. Cucumbers are an excellent antidote to our modern toxic environments. Cucumbers are high in the mineral silica, which is needed for healthy skin, connective tissue, hair, and bones. They also contain vitamin C, potassium, magnesium, and fibre. Choose only organic cucumbers because traditionally grown varieties are sprayed with pesticides and the skin is usually waxed, which may "lock in" these harmful toxins. The cucumber's plant sterols and many of its other nutrients are found in the skin.

Flaxseeds/Flaxseed Oil—Packed with anti-inflammatory, anti-pain, and health-promoting Omega 3 fatty acids (the ones most people aren't getting enough of), ground flaxseeds and flaxseed oil are excellent additions to your diet. The seeds also contain a high amount of fibre to help keep you regular. They also bind to toxins to escort them out of your body. Research shows that the daily consumption of Omega 3s from flax can reduce pain and inflammation, including in arthritics. Additionally, scientists have also discovered that Omega 3s aid bone health. Omega 3s even help to protect the brain against toxins. Their anti-inflammatory effects make them helpful in the prevention and treatment of arteriosclerosis as well. I suspect that over time, researchers will identify even more health benefits of Omega 3s since you may recall from our earlier discussion that your body needs adequate amounts of Omega 3 fatty acids to ensure the proper function of your cells, tissues, and organs. Avoid cooking with flaxseeds or flaxseed oil. Instead, add either the ground seeds or oil to already cooked foods or salads. I toss a tablespoon of the ground seeds into smoothies for a nutritious energy drink. Keep both the ground seeds and oil stored in your refrigerator.

Ginger—Fresh ginger offers so many health benefits while adding a wonderful taste to so many foods that you'll want to eat this Life Force Gold Food on a regular basis. Ginger has been shown to be superior to non-steroidal anti-inflammatory drugs (NSAIDs) at alleviating pain and inflammation. Unlike NSAIDs that work on one level to reduce pain, ginger works on two: 1) it blocks the formation of substances in the body that are linked to pain; and 2) it has antioxidant properties that break down inflammation.[9] As you now know, inflammation is linked to most chronic illnesses and premature aging. Additionally, ginger stimulates circulation, reduces the stickiness of the blood, reduces cholesterol levels, aids digestion and nausea, and is helpful for respiratory infections. I make a pot of fresh ginger tea on an almost daily basis especially on cold days by chopping a two- to three-inch piece of ginger root and simmering it on the stove for 10 minutes in 4 to 5 cups of water. Add a little stevia or a touch of honey, and you'll enjoy a delicious tea and your body will enjoy many health rewards. You can also add finely chopped ginger to stir-fries, soups, stews, or curries, or sauté ginger matchsticks and toss on a green salad as in my Life Force Salad (see page 244).

Grapes—Purple or red grapes are an excellent source of the phytonutrient quercetin, which has been shown to prevent depression, improve mental functioning, and lessen breathing problems linked to asthma. Purple or red grapes also contain the phytonutrient resveratrol, which has many health benefits, including atherosclerosis prevention and increasing longevity. Ellagic acid is another valuable phytonutrient found in grapes. Research shows that this phytonutrient has anti-cancer properties. Grapes are also a good source of the mineral boron, which is needed for bone health and hormonal production, particularly in post-menopausal women.

Grapefruit—Not only are grapefruits one of nature's best cholesterol fighters when eaten daily, they are also rich in pectin—a type of fibre that binds to excess cholesterol and toxins, particularly heavy metals, and escorts them out of the body. Grapefruits are also rich in the phytonutrient limonene, which has valuable anti-cancer properties and has been shown to reduce mammary tumours in rats. Pink grapefruits contain lycopene, which helps protect against bladder, cervical, and pancreatic cancer as well. And I'm sure you don't need me to tell you that grapefruits are an excellent source of vitamin C—an important antioxidant to help conquer the effects of stress and aging.

Kiwis—Originally called *souris végétale* by the French, which means "vegetable mouse," this fuzzy little fruit was renamed by New Zealanders and is now known as kiwi or kiwi fruit. Abundant in vitamin C, other antioxidants, and Omega 3 fatty acids, eating kiwi is an excellent way to boost immunity and strengthen brain power. Kiwis also have a fair amount of potassium and fibre. Kiwi also contains the important phytonutrient lutein that helps prevent cataracts and macular degeneration by maintaining eye health. While there are many enzymes found in kiwis, they contain a particularly valuable one called actinidin, which helps to digest proteins in food. Peel off the fuzzy skin, and slice or chop and add to fruit salads or top a green salad with some kiwi slices for a unique and delicious salad.

Lemons—Containing over 22 anti-cancer compounds, lemons and their freshly squeezed juice are valuable contributors to disease-prevention and great health. One of these compounds is limonene—a naturally occurring oil that slows or halts the growth of cancer tumours in animals. Rich in both vitamin C and flavonoids that work in conjunction with this vitamin for greater health-enhancing properties, lemons pack a serious punch against infection. Fresh lemon juice added to a large glass of water in the morning is not only a great natural energy booster, but a liver detoxifier and body chemistry balancer. I juice a whole lemon and add it to water every morning and wait ½ hour before eating breakfast to boost my life force.

Lettuce—Greens of virtually all kinds are among nature's greatest Life Force Gold Foods. Packed with vitamins, minerals, chlorophyll, phytonutrients, and enzymes, lettuces will assume a priority place in your life force diet. Forget iceberg lettuce though, since it is primarily water and contains few nutrients. Instead, choose greens that actually live up to their name—the darker the colour, the more intense the nutrients. Romaine lettuce is particularly good, with its high beta carotene, fibre, and potassium content. But don't overlook mixtures of baby greens like "mesclun," "spring mix," or other lettuce blends. Most of them contain high amounts of calcium and magnesium needed for strong bones, muscles, and a relaxed nervous system. Eat at least one large salad with Life Force Gold lettuce every day to maximize your health and disease-fighting potential. Just avoid dressing your greens with a high-sugar, nutrient-deprived, preservative-filled store-bought dressing when it is so easy and fast to make delicious ones at home (check out some of my recipes in Chapter 9).

Limes—In addition to the high amount of vitamin C found in limes, they contain a particular flavonoid called flavonol glycosides, which have been shown to stop cell division in cancer cells. Additionally, this flavonoid has demonstrated antibiotic effects, particularly in research involving several villages in West Africa where cholera epidemics occurred. Adding lime juice to the preparation of foods appeared to have a protective effect against the contraction of cholera.[10] Other research shows that lime juice seems to affect the body's immune system cells to aid in their decision to divide or die—a decision immune cells face regularly to avoid the unhealthy division of diseased cells like cancerous ones. Squeeze fresh lime juice over a salad, use in a freshly made salad dressing, add to water, or enjoy in my delicious guacamole recipe found in the recipe section at the back of this book.

Mangoes—As delicious as they are nutritious, if you're not already eating mangoes in your diet you might want to reconsider. Bursting with beta carotene (the plant form of vitamin A), vitamin C, potassium, and fibre, mangoes deserve their rightful place in your life force diet. Complete with energy-boosting and stress-managing minerals like iron, potassium, and magnesium, mangoes are an important food addition to our fast-paced and hectic lives. Mangoes are also rich in phytonutrients like quercetin that helps protect against respiratory problems, alleviate asthma, and reduce allergic reactions. Mangoes are also rich sources of enzymes that improve digestion, detoxify the intestines, and improve overall health. Because they contain the amino acid tryptophan, which is readily converted in the body to an important mood-balancing hormone called serotonin, mangoes can help lift your spirits, reduce anxiety, and lessen depression. Look for mangoes that have mostly turned yellow and yield slightly to touch. Make two lengthwise slices along the sides of the mango to remove the pit and peel to reveal its juicy yellow-gold flesh. Add this part to smoothies, atop a salad, or diced as part of a chutney accompaniment to curries.

Olive Oil—An essential part of Mediterranean diets, olive oil deserves a place in the life force diet as well. Olive oil appears to reduce harmful cholesterol while increasing beneficial cholesterol levels, making it helpful to lessen the risk of heart disease. It is still wise to use sparingly since it is a highly rich food. Choose an organic, first-pressed, extra virgin olive oil wherever possible. Use it to cook with (although never heat it above about 325 degrees Fahrenheit, which is this oil's smoke point and after which it is no longer healthy to ingest), make dressings and marinades, and to drizzle on veggies. Research shows that marinating food in olive oil and lemon juice reduces the potential for carcinogen formation in grilled food by up to 99 percent.

Oranges—I would bet that oranges are North Americans' favourite fruit and it's a well-deserved title. This healthy fruit not only contains vitamin C, folate, and potassium, it also contains a particular type of fibre called pectin that is especially good at binding heavy metals like lead and mercury in your body to escort them out in your bowel movements so they are less likely to cause brain or neurological damage. Additionally, they contain the phytonutrients limonene and polyphenols. Polyphenols assist with weight loss, particularly burning abdominal fat. Research shows that oranges help ward off cancer, diabetes, stroke, and many other serious health conditions. I have included a delicious salad called the life force salad that includes fresh oranges in the recipe section of this book. It's important to ingest foods high in vitamin C, like oranges, lemons, grapefruit, red peppers, etc. on a regular basis since vitamin C is water soluble. In your body, that means it is used up and any excess is excreted in your urine and not stored for later use.

Papayas—Papayas are not only rich with beta carotene, as their orange-reddish flesh would indicate, but they are also enzyme powerhouses. They also contain high amounts of vitamin C.

Ripe papayas contain an enzyme, papain, which helps to break down protein in your body. When not working directly on food, papain helps to reduce inflammation in the body, making you less vulnerable to pain, joint inflammation, other types of inflammation in the body, and the effects of aging. Soothing to the digestive tract and helpful to alleviate gas and toxic waste in the intestines, as well as to balance good bacteria, papaya is an important Life Force Gold Food.

Peaches—Growing up in one of Canada's "fruit belts," I was fortunate enough to have a peach tree in our backyard. Every day during peach season, I would race home from school to enjoy the juicy and delectable fruits nature had ripened overnight. I would frequently eat three or more even at the age of only five or six. As long as fresh peaches were in season, candy held little appeal, which is good because unlike candy, peaches are loaded with beta carotene, fibre, natural energy-boosting sugars, and some potassium as well. Add fresh peaches to smoothies, blend alongside frozen peeled bananas instead of ice cream, or top a plate of greens with them for a delicious addition to lunch or dinner.

Pears—Pears are a good source of vitamins C and K, and the mineral potassium. Like apples, pears are high in a specific type of fibre called pectin, which binds to heavy metals and other toxins in the body and helps to escort them out. Pears also improve "transit time" in the intestines—the time it takes for foods to be digested, assimilated, and the remaining waste to be removed, making pears beneficial for anyone who suffers from chronic constipation, which is almost everyone. If you're having fewer than two or three healthy bowel movements daily, start eating pears instead of sweets. Pears tend to be well tolerated by almost everyone.

Pineapples—Another enzyme powerhouse, when ripe, this delicious fruit contains high amounts of the enzyme bromelain, which helps improve digestion, eliminate inflammation, and lessen pain linked to inflammation in the body. That is why pineapple is such a great food for people suffering from arthritis, and other types of pain and inflammation disorders. Bromelain also helps to thin mucus in the body, making it helpful for bronchitis, sinus problems, and asthma. Bromelain helps with high blood pressure and heart disease. Plus, when pineapples taste so good, who wouldn't want to get more bromelain in his or her diet? Eat them on their own, diced in a fruit chutney or fruit salad, add slices to a green salad for a real treat, or add to a smoothie.

Plums—I grew up in an Italian district where people grew all kinds of fruit trees, including Italian plum trees. When plums were in season, the generous Italians I worked with or went to school with would bring bags or boxes of extra plums to share with others. That was my first introduction to plums and it led me to develop a real appreciation for these yummy Life Force Gold Foods. While plums contain vitamin A, B2, C, iron, potassium, and fibre, their true strength appears to lie in their phytonutrient content. Plums contain the unique phytonutrients called neochlorogenic and chlorogenic acid, both of which are types of phenols and are well-researched potent antioxidants. These compounds are particularly effective at neutralizing a type of free radical called superoxide anion radical, which is a serious threat to healthy cells and tissues, including brain neurons. The phytonutrients in plums have a protective effect on fatty components of cells, including brain and nervous system cells and are a powerful ally against free radical damage. Enjoy them diced in a fruit salad, blended with frozen berries for a delicious smoothie or fruit ice cream, or sliced on top of a green salad.

Pomegranates—These delicious fruits offer more than just incredible taste, they are anti-aging and anti-cancer powerhouses. Studies in the laboratory on pomegranate juice's effects against cancer as well as on men with prostate cancer have shown tremendous promise. The antioxidants and/or phytonutrients in pomegranates also appear to interact with the body's genetic material for protection. Pomegranates are packed with vitamin C and the phytonutrients polyphenols and ellagic acid. You can eat them fresh as a Life Force Gold Food or drink unsweetened bottled pomegranate juice devoid of preservatives as a Life Force Silver Food. For the latter, I recommend diluting 1 part water to 1 part pomegranate juice to avoid blood sugar spikes and crashes. I sometimes use a splash of pomegranate juice in my salad dressing for incredible anti-aging benefits and to jazz up a plate of greens. I also throw a handful of pomegranate berries on top for an extra kick. Yum!

Raspberries—My grandparents grew a huge fruit and vegetable garden. Whenever I visited them in the summer, I quickly disappeared into the several rows of raspberry bushes to see if they were ripe yet. And, oh the joy I experienced if they were ready to eat! My grandmother would give me a couple of baskets to fill. For every raspberry that I put into the basket at least one or two others would find their way into my mouth. It would take me a while to fill the baskets but I had no problem filling my stomach with these ruby red bursts of flavour. Raspberries are still one of my favourite fruits and they both satisfy a desire for something sweet and remind me of some sweet childhood memories. Raspberries contain vitamin C, potassium, and fibre. In Chinese medicine they are used to improve liver and kidney function as well as to cleanse the blood of toxins. They are also used to treat anemia and encourage labour in childbirth. Raspberries, like other berries, contain an important compound that is 10 times more effective at alleviating inflammation than Aspirin. Containing the phytonutrient ellagic acid, raspberries can help protect against pollutants found in cigarette smoke, and processed foods, and may neutralize some cancer-causing substances before they can damage healthy cells. They're delicious on their own, in a fruit salad, in a smoothie, or on top of a green salad.

Spinach—Not just for Popeye anymore, spinach is high in iron, calcium, beta carotene (which turns into vitamin A in your body), and vitamin K, which is important for bone and blood health. Additionally, chlorophyll, which gives spinach leaves their green colour, is a powerful blood cleanser. Also high in the phytonutrient neoxanthin, which has been shown to support prostate health, spinach truly is an excellent Life Force Gold Food for both men and women. Spinach is high in other phytonutrients like lutein and zeaxanthin, which are excellent for strengthening your eyes and vision and helpful in preventing disorders of the eyes like macular degeneration and cataracts. The rest of your body benefits from the spinach's glutathione and alpha lipoic acid content. Both of these nutrients play a critical role in detoxifying harmful chemicals you may have been exposed to in your food, air, and water. Glutathione even helps prevent tumours from becoming cancerous. Alpha lipoic acid has antioxidant properties that are even stronger than vitamins C and E. Research from the University of California at Berkeley indicates that it may assist in preventing diabetes and heart disease. What makes this nutrient special, though, is that it crosses the blood-brain barrier to access the delicate brain where it may help prevent free radical damage that leads to brain disease or stroke.[11]

Strawberries—Every June when strawberries burst into gardens and markets across the continent, I am reminded of my strawberry-picking expeditions as a child with my dad and sister. My mom agreed to make dozens of pies or fresh jam if we'd pick the strawberries needed. Well, that was all the incentive I needed to spend some serious time in the massive strawberry patches in the countryside near where I lived. Nowadays, I try to eat fresh strawberries to benefit from both the nutrients and the enzymes they contain. More than delicious, when it comes to disease prevention, these babies pack a serious punch. Not only do eight strawberries contain more vitamin C than an orange, they are antioxidant powerhouses! Whether you want to evade heart disease, arthritis, memory loss, or cancer, these berries have proven their ability to help. Plus, they're just so easy to get into your diet on a regular basis: Add fresh or frozen strawberries to smoothies, shakes, or blender "juices," top whole-grain, dairy-free pancakes with fresh strawberries, or just enjoy them on their own.

Walnuts—Walnuts are an important addition to your diet since they offer high amounts of Omega 3 fatty acids needed to protect your brain, maintain a healthy immune system, balance moods, and lessen pain and inflammation in your body. Chinese medicine practitioners have believed for many years that walnuts (which look like little brains!) are beneficial for brain health. Modern scientists are proving them right—their Omega 3 fatty acid content makes them especially great for your brain. What's more, walnuts contain vitamins B6 and E and minerals like magnesium and potassium. These minerals are important to ward off the effects of stress, strengthen your nervous system, and reduce pain. I toss them on top of salads or chop them and stir them into my Vanilla Ice Cream recipe, which you'll find in the recipe section. For years I believed that I couldn't stand the taste of walnuts, but when I tried fresh, refrigerated walnuts from a health food store, I realized I loved them! If you have had walnuts in the past and didn't like them, give them another try and buy them from the refrigerator of a health food store. That awful taste that I couldn't stand came from the rancid oils in walnuts that are old or commercially processed with heat.

Watermelon—Tomatoes aren't the only food that contains high amounts of the phytonutrient lycopene, known for its prostate-protecting, anti-aging, and disease-thwarting powers. Additionally, watermelon is a refreshing cleansing food that, due to its high vitamin C, beta carotene, and glutathione content, helps to remove toxins from your blood and improve detoxification in your liver. I enjoy watermelon juice by simply removing the green outer layer and adding chunks of the pink flesh to a blender and blending until smooth. Watermelon juice is a perfect thirst quencher for a hot summer day. I also love watermelon in fruit salad or as a snack throughout the day.[12]

7

Give Your Life Force a Boost

EATING Life Force Gold and Silver Foods is the fastest way to great health, balanced weight, energy, and vitality. By adding a few natural supplements and lifestyle additions, you'll speed the whole process along and give it another boost. Let's take a look at the best supplements to add to your life force diet for optimum health and well-being. Since I'm not a fan of popping handfuls of vitamins and minerals, I encourage you to add the following carefully selected supplements to your diet: a broad-spectrum digestive enzyme, co-enzyme Q10, probiotics, greens, and Cellfood®. You'll notice that the enzymes, probiotics, and greens are basically food supplements, meaning that they are concentrated from foods. Cellfood® is a liquid supplement that requires only 8 drops in water or juice and is easily absorbed. And, as you'll soon learn, coenzyme Q10 is necessary for every function in your body and is an excellent way to supercharge your health and energy.

Supplementing Your Life Force

You may recall our earlier discussion about the enzymes found in uncooked Life Force Gold Foods. These potent super healers have just the right amount of enzymes to digest themselves. Your body must manufacture the enzymes needed to break down any cooked foods in your diet, including Life Force Silver Foods. Creating these enzymes requires a fair amount of energy, particularly from your liver and pancreas—the two organs situated on the right and left sides respectively of your upper abdomen, just under your lower ribs. By taking a high-potency digestive enzyme with every meal you can improve digestion while increasing your energy and the absorption of the nutrients found in the foods you eat. Through increased nutrient absorption, every cell can function more effectively. Reducing the need for energy from the heavy task of digestion means it can be reallocated elsewhere—this also has the result of improving every function in your body.

How to Choose a Good Digestive Enzyme Supplement

As you learned earlier, foods contain enough enzymes in their unadulterated state to help your body digest them. While you will experience the profound healing effects of eating a diet high in enzyme-rich foods, sometimes your body needs more, particularly after many years of abuse and neglect from feeding it nutrient- and enzyme-deprived foods. By taking a digestive enzyme supplement, you can support your body's own digestive processes. And, remember, that means you'll be supporting your body's ability to extract all the critical nutrients you need from the foods you eat to ensure healthy cells and tissues.

By taking digestive enzyme supplements with meals or any time you are consuming food, you reduce your body's need to manufacture its own digestive enzymes, thereby decreasing the energy spent on digestion, which can be reallocated toward healing and disease prevention. This simple life force booster can help you feel better than ever and may even increase your life span!

My clients are always astounded when they start taking digestive enzyme supplements, particularly if they are accustomed to suffering from bloating and indigestion with or soon after meals.

So how do you choose a good-quality digestive enzyme supplement? Well, there are numerous factors to consider. A high-quality digestive enzyme should

1. Not contain any genetically modified ingredients—if the label doesn't tell you this information, the product may contain these potentially harmful GMOs.
2. Be manufactured by a reputable company. You may need to conduct some research on the manufacturing practices of the products in which you are interested. Unfortunately there are wide degrees of variation in quality between health products. I am routinely frustrated by the lack of quality of many health supplements. Whenever consumer product tests are conducted, only a small percentage of products actually contain the ingredients the manufacturers claim they do, so do some research to find out if the products you are choosing are reputable.
3. Be devoid of colours, sugars, artificial flavours, or other harmful ingredients that can cause health risks. I once had a client come with a large plastic bag full of all the supplements she purchased at a major retail outlet. When I explored the ingredients on the labels, I spotted plentiful amounts of sugars and even colours. She was shocked when I pointed out these suspect ingredients. These harmful substances have no place in your food, and they certainly do not belong in your supplements.
4. Contain a broad spectrum of enzymes. In other words, it should contain **amylase** to break down carbohydrates, **cellulase** to digest fibre, **lipase** to break down fats, and **protease** to digest proteins. If you haven't been able to wean yourself off dairy products, you'll also want to obtain an enzyme product that contains lactase to digest the milk sugars as well.

5. Be from vegetarian sources if you are a vegetarian. Many enzyme products are from animal sources (I'll tell you more about them momentarily) and that is fine, but if you strive to be completely vegetarian for ethical, religious, or other reasons, you'll want to be sure your enzyme supplement is devoid of ingredients like pancreatin, trypsin, and chymotrypsin.

6. Ideally, contain the minerals and nutrients that aid with the functioning of enzymes. Your body requires specific nutrients that work synergistically with enzymes and ensure they can perform their important functions. Try to choose an enzyme product that contains the following nutrients: bromine, calcium, iodine, iron, magnesium, molybdenum, phosphorus, potassium, selenium, sulphur, and zinc.

Ignite Your Life Force

STEP 23   Supercharge Your Digestion with Enzymes

By supplementing with a broad-spectrum digestive enzyme, you'll free up your body's energy for other bodily functions rather than for manufacturing digestive enzymes. This is especially important since cooking destroys the enzymes in food, which means that your body must compensate with its own digestive enzymes. Supplementing with digestive enzymes lessens the burden on your body. But be sure to choose an enzyme supplement that contains a wide range of enzymes, including

- Amylase
- Cellulase
- Invertase
- Lipase
- Malt Diastase
- Protease

A wide range of enzymes helps to ensure that all components of the foods you eat are digested, including the starches, sugars, fats, proteins, and fibre. While dairy foods are not part of the life force diet, if you are still eating them, you will also want to ensure your digestive enzyme product also contains lactase to digest the milk sugars.

What about Stomach Acid and Enzymes?

Frequently biochemists like to argue that enzymes are completely destroyed by the acidity of the stomach, regardless of their source. Painting with a rather broad brush, these people propose that all food enzymes and digestive enzyme supplements are rendered useless by hydrochloric acid found in the stomach.

Here's why that argument is false. Typically people who claim that enzymes are killed by stomach acid cite the pH (highly acidic) of the stomach combined with enzymes' sensitivity to pH as the reason. However, not all enzymes are the same. While some enzymes prefer a more alkaline environment, some do their best work in acidic environments. Certain enzymes like animal-source ones (pancreatin, trypsin, and chymotrypsin, for example) are especially sensitive to acidity. They work in an alkaline medium. You may have heard of enteric coated enzymes. Usually these types of enzymes are coated to ensure that they pass through the stomach virtually untouched until they reach the small intestine (which is alkaline) where they are released to do their work.

However, research conducted by the organization founded by the father of enzyme research, Dr. Edward Howell, found that most plant-based enzymes like those found in Life Force Gold Foods are active in an acidic environment. In this study researchers conducted four different tests: 1) on the meal without digestive enzymes under ideal digestive conditions; 2) on the meal with a digestive enzyme blend under ideal digestive conditions; 3) on the meal without the digestive enzyme blend with 70 percent reduced digestive secretions; and 4) on the meal with the digestive enzymes under impaired digestion. They collected samples at various times during the digestive process to analyze carbohydrate and protein digestion. The enzymes improved the digestion of both carbs and proteins under both impaired and ideal digestive conditions. Actually, glucose availability (the measure of how well the carbohydrates were broken down into simple sugars) was increased 400 percent in the ideal digestive system and 700 percent in the impaired digestive system. The researchers concluded that the enzymes survive the acidity of the stomach![1]

But, research aside, anyone who suffers from digestive troubles and has ever taken a quality plant-based enzyme supplement along with meals knows that most of these enzymes survive the stomach acid. They feel less bloating, gas, and digestive discomfort when taking them.

When to Add Pancreatic Enzymes

There are times when some people may benefit from taking pancreatic enzymes along with plant enzymes and meals. You may recall our earlier discussion about the important role of the pancreas in manufacturing enzymes to assist with digestion (as well as to produce insulin). If you are suffering from an inflamed, sluggish, or malfunctioning pancreas, you may want to add a pancreatic enzyme supplement to your diet, in addition to the broad spectrum digestive enzyme supplement mentioned above. It's best to consult with a natural health practitioner specializing in enzyme therapy to determine if you need to support your pancreas's enzyme production.

The Nutrient That Assists Every Cell in Your Body

Needed by every cell in your body, the important nutrient Coenzyme Q10 plays a critical role in ensuring you have the energy your body needs to heal, maintain a strong immune system, and fight the cellular damage linked with aging. Unfortunately, CoQ10, as it is also called, naturally decreases as we age, so it is beneficial to replenish your body's supplies.

Coenzyme Q10, like other coenzymes, is an assistant to the thousands of enzymes in your body. It helps to transport chemicals and nutrients to enzymes where the enzymes can do their work. Every cell in your body requires CoQ10 to produce adequate energy to perform its many functions. Without adequate amounts, cells and processes in your body simply don't have the energy they need to perform their functions.

Supplementing with coenzyme Q10 helps to jump-start energy production in your cells and increase your overall energy and stamina. It also helps to boost heart health by strengthening your heart and cardiovascular system, acts as a potent antioxidant and protector against free radicals linked to cellular and organ damage, reduces the effects of aging, helps promote healthy blood pressure, and boosts your immune system. What's more, CoQ10 increases the longevity of other antioxidant nutrients to help them continue protecting your body for longer periods. CoQ10 also helps ensure that your brain has sufficient cellular energy to perform its important and myriad tasks. And it helps to normalize weight!

It is especially important to supplement with coenzyme Q10 if you take statin drugs since these medications rely on the same biochemical pathway to lower cholesterol as your body does to produce CoQ10, putting you at further risk of insufficient quantities.

As with all supplements you should only purchase from companies with strict quality control practices and whose supplements are devoid of synthetic or genetically modified ingredients. The most active form of CoQ10 is ubiquinol: It can sometimes be difficult to find, but it is worth the effort.

Ignite Your Life Force

> **STEP 24** **Jump-start Your Cells' Energy Centres**
>
> Since CoQ10 is needed for almost every function of your body, especially to power the energy centres of your cells, and because it tends to wane as we get older, I suggest supplementing with this important coenzyme. As you may recall, coenzymes help to ensure that enzymes can function properly so they are critical to ensure strong enzyme power in your body. Ideally, I suggest taking 50 to 100 mg of CoQ10 daily along with meals and your digestive enzyme supplement to help ensure maximum absorption of this important nutrient.

Pro Power

Over time probiotics, the beneficial bacteria that normally reside in your small and large intestines, can wear out. They can also become vulnerable to destruction by imbalanced populations of harmful microbes in the intestines that can be the result of excess sugar consumption, antibiotic use, and many other factors. Because probiotics are so important to overall health, as well as necessary to produce certain enzymes, including cellulose, lactase, protease, and amylase—which are necessary for healthy digestion and a strong immune system—it's important to replenish your body's stores with a probiotic supplement. Choose one that contains a wide variety of bacteria strains, including *Lactobacillus acidophilus* (also called *L. acidophilus*), *Lactobacillus bifidus*, *Bacillus subtillus*, *Lactobacillus casei*, *Lactobacillus bulgaris*, *Lactobacillus plantarum*, *Lactobacillus rhamnosus*, *Lactobacillus salivarius*, *Lactobacillus longum*, *Lactobacillus lactis*, *Lactobacillus F-19*, and *Bifidobacterium bifidum*.

Be aware that many of these bacteria do not survive the acidity of the stomach, so it is important to choose ones that are enteric coated, if possible. Don't worry if you can't find a supplement that contains all of the above strains. Since each strain tends to have a special role in the body, the more strains you can find in a particular supplement, typically the better. But it's far more important to ensure that the bacteria remain intact by the time they reach the intestines and enteric-coated probiotics often help in this regard.

Ignite Your Life Force

STEP 25 Power Up with Probiotics

Replenish your body's natural healthy bacteria levels by adding a broad-spectrum probiotic supplement to your diet. Ideally, look for one in which the capsules are enteric coated and contain *L. acidophilus, L. bifidus, B. subtilus, L. casei, L. bulgaris, L. plantarum, L. rhamnosus, L. salivarius, L. longum, L. lactis, L. F-19,* and *B. bifidum.* Take two capsules on an empty stomach.

Superfood for Super Health

In the first few chapters, we discussed the important role that vitamins and minerals play in ensuring healthy cells and in support of enzyme production and utilization in your body. One of the best ways to ensure that you are getting adequate vitamins and minerals is by supplementing your diet with a green food supplement made from barley grass juice, wheat grass juice, chlorella, or another "green food." These supplements typically provide a broad range of nutrients in a form that is recognizable to the body, and therefore more usable. Be sure to check the label to avoid products full of sugars or other unwanted ingredients. And try to find a supplement that is processed using low temperatures and that guarantees the enzymes remain intact. That way, you'll be boosting your enzyme intake at the same time.

These supplements also supply the phytonutrient chlorophyll, which provides plants with their green colour. In the body, chlorophyll helps to balance your body's pH to be more alkaline (most of us are too acidic), helps strengthen your blood, and boosts energy.

Some green food supplements come in tablet or capsule form, which is fine if that's how you prefer them. But they truly are better when ingested in a powder form. It's easy enough to do by adding them to juices or smoothies. They actually add a slightly sweet taste. Some people are turned off by the colour they turn juices and smoothies, but are usually surprised that the taste is still pleasant.

If you are diabetic you may want to supplement your diet with vitamin A. Typically the body can turn beta carotene found in green food supplements or in your daily diet into vitamin A, but this function is frequently impaired in people with diabetes. If you are diabetic and choose to supplement with vitamin A, look for a supplement that offers 5000 IU (international units) of vitamin A. Do not increase your dosage without first seeking the advice of a qualified health professional since vitamin A is stored in the body and over time can build up excessively.

Ignite Your Life Force

STEP 26 Increase Your Green Power

Green food supplements like barley grass, wheat grass juice, chlorella, alfalfa, and spirulina are packed with vitamins, minerals, and phytonutrients. Choose one that guarantees the enzymes are still intact (the product should have been processed at extremely low temperatures and most say on the label if they were) for even better nutritional support. Start slowly by adding a teaspoon to your daily diet each day of the first week you take a green food supplement. Then increase to two teaspoons, either at once or taken in two drinks during the day. After another week, increase to a tablespoon daily.

Cellfood®

Cellfood® is a unique cell-oxygenating liquid formula that delivers 78 trace minerals, 34 enzymes, 17 amino acids, and electrolytes, and increases the bioavailability of oxygen to the body. It is readily absorbed by the body at the cellular level, making a wealth of nutrients available to your cells for optimum healing. Unlike other oxygen products I've tried, Cellfood® delivers the oxygen slowly, thereby preventing free radical damage. Cellfood® also helps normalize an acidic pH of the body, which is integral to proper detoxification and healing. It also assists with energy and boosts the immune system.

Ignite Your Life Force

> **STEP 27** Recharge Your Cells
>
> Take 8 drops of Cellfood® three times per day in a glass of pure water or juice to give your body trace minerals, enzymes, oxygen, and other nutrients needed for optimum health and well-being.

Other Supplements

Does that mean that you should only ever take the five supplements I suggested? No. There are certain health conditions or times in our lives that would benefit from other supplements. Of course, you should consult a nutrition expert to select the best ones for you. I strongly suggest that you avoid just taking whatever supplement happens to be "in fashion" at any given time simply because it is touted in articles as a cure-all. Such approaches to health give no consideration to biochemical individuality—those factors that make our bodies unique. While the vast majority of substances needed by our bodies are the same from one person to the next, the precise amounts of particular nutrients may vary between individuals. The ones I have selected are essential to almost everyone, but you may feel the need to add other supplements depending on your health circumstances, genetic predispositions, lifestyle, or other determining factors.

Go for Your Life Force Supercharged

You may be wondering how you can fit these supplements into your daily regime. It's actually much easier than you might think. And once you get into a regular daily program, it will become natural for you over time. Here's a possible way to include the supplements into your day:

- Before breakfast: Add 8 drops Cellfood® in a large glass of water with freshly squeezed lemon juice to help rehydrate your cells quickly. Take a digestive enzyme supplement at this time.
- With breakfast: Take Coenzyme Q10 with your breakfast and add your green supplement to a breakfast smoothie. Not having a breakfast smoothie? Don't worry, just take your green supplement in juice or a smoothie later in the day.
- Half an hour before lunch: Add another 8 drops of Cellfood® in water or juice and take your digestive enzyme supplement.
- Half an hour before dinner: Add 8 drops of Cellfood® in water or juice and take another digestive enzyme supplement.
- Before bed: Take 2 capsules of probiotics with a small amount of water.

The Life Force Lifestyle

It's also important to support your body's natural functions through exercise. That doesn't mean you have to head to the gym if that's not your thing. Exercise can take many forms of physical activity. Choose whatever type that is fun for you: walking, cycling, hiking, soccer, running, hockey, kayaking, or any other form of activity that gets your blood pumping.

Our bodies were made to move. They were not made to sit at a desk all day, to slouch in front of the television all night, or play video games all weekend. Activity helps to increase blood flow to cells and organs, delivering much-needed oxygen to help them dispel wastes and function better. Our muscles need to be used to obtain fresh oxygenated blood. Every cell, tissue, organ, and organ system in your body benefits from exercise, and actually *needs* exercise to function properly.

Our lymphatic system—an extensive network of vessels, nodes, glands, and fluid—needs exercise to work properly. Though the lymphatic system contains three times more fluid than blood, it has no heart to pump it. It relies on exercise. This system is responsible for gathering toxins throughout our bodies and moving them back to be dumped into the bloodstream. At that point, the major detoxification organs like the kidneys and liver filter the toxins from the blood for elimination from the body. If you're not getting sufficient activity, your lymphatic system will allow toxins to build up. You'll feel sluggish, experience pain, and may even observe cellulite and fat deposits. And that's because toxins are building up in your body. You may even feel like you're wading through swamp water, because that's what's happening in your lymphatic system!

Exercise also helps keep toxins eliminated from your intestines, which, as you learned earlier, would otherwise be absorbed back into your bloodstream through the walls of the intestines. Regular activity helps keep you regular.

As part of the life force diet, it's important to get sufficient activity. Be sure to take a brisk walk for at least 20 minutes daily. Did you know that walking just 20 minutes three times a week is proven to increase energy levels by 20 percent and decrease fatigue by 65 percent?[2]

Or choose another form of cardiovascular activity if you prefer to do something else. If you need variety in your life, walk one day, bike another, jump rope another day, or whatever else suits your activity style. Just get moving.

> ### *Summary of Supplementing the Life Force Diet—Weeks 1 to 3*
>
> 1. Supercharge your digestion with a broad-spectrum enzyme supplement taken before or with every meal.
> 2. Jump-start your cell's energy centres by supplementing with 50 to 100 mg of CoQ10 daily taken with food.
> 3. Power up with probiotics by taking a broad-spectrum probiotic supplement on an empty stomach every day.
> 4. Increase your green power by adding a green food powder such as barley grass, wheat grass juice, chlorella, alfalfa, or spirulina to juice or smoothies. Take 1 teaspoon daily for the first week, increase to 2 teaspoons for week two, and then increase to 1 tablespoon for week three and thereafter.
> 5. Recharge your cells by adding 8 drops of Cellfood® in water or juice three times daily.

The Life Force Diet isn't hard; it just takes commitment to your health and yourself. And the minimal effort it takes will reward you with vibrant good looks, super immunity against disease, and renewed energy and vitality. You are worth it—not just for three weeks but for life!

PART THREE

Creating Luscious
Life Force Recipes

8

Preparing Your Life Force Banquet

NOW that you've learned about the miracle healing and weight-balancing properties of the life force diet, you may be wondering how to get started preparing delicious life force food.

The most common complaint I hear from people wanting to feel healthier is that they don't have time to prepare healthy food, it's too much work, or it costs too much to eat healthily. The reality is that with some added knowledge it takes very little time, effort, or money to eat well and the result is greater energy to do all the other things you want to do. So, in essence, preparing food and eating the life force way increases your time.

In this chapter you will learn how to equip your kitchen for the best results, which low-cost tools are essential and which ones are just helpful additions, how to stock your pantry, how to sprout, how to cook grains, a table for using herbs suitable for the herbal novice and expert alike, how to travel the life force way, and how to make the life force diet work for your family. Armed with this information, you'll find that sticking to the life force diet is easy for life. And you'll be amazed at how simple, inexpensive, and rewarding life force eating can be, even if you're on the road, have young children, have an intense career, or just have a busy life. Isn't that just about everyone these days?

Equipping the Life Force Kitchen

While you really don't need any special equipment to prepare your life force banquet, there are a few handy items to add to make following the life force diet easy for life. But don't give up the whole program if you don't have these items or don't have the money to purchase them. You can still do marvellously with nothing more than a knife, cutting board, pan, and a bowl or two. Because of the important role of salads in the life force diet, you may wish to get a good salad spinner, since they can make light work of cleaning and drying greens. You can purchase a good-quality one for about $20 or less. You can add a juicer, food processor, blender as you are able, to minimize the effort and maximize results. I also suggest a good-quality ice cream maker, for delicious and healthy treats.

Food Processor

A food processor makes light work of chopping, mincing, grating, slicing, and mixing. In seconds, it can complete what might take many minutes to do, thereby making it a snap to complete life force recipes when you're short on time. There are many good-quality ones on the market at affordable prices.

Juice It Up

The idea of juicing fresh fruits and vegetables first started with a man named Norman Walker. Born in 1875, he was recovering from health problems in the French countryside. While observing the women in the kitchen peeling carrots, he noticed how moist the vegetables were beneath the skin. He had the idea that grinding them for the juice would help him recover his health, which proved accurate. Later, he moved to California, where he and a medical doctor friend opened a juice bar, concocting fresh juices for specific health conditions—and the fresh juice craze had begun in North America.

Walker's belief that fresh juices could help heal countless health conditions has been upheld by many health centres throughout North America that still treat people primarily with nutrient- and life force–packed juices. But you don't need to visit one of these health clinics to start restoring your body's health, vitality, and life force immediately. With minimal effort you can juice at home.

While a juicer is not an essential part of the life force diet, it is a great addition and is highly recommended. Freshly made vegetable and fruit juices pack a tonne of nutrition in every sip; they are also loaded with enzymes, which increase your life force energy.

There are many different kinds of juicers, ranging from $40 to over $1000. While the more expensive ones may offer superior quality and nutrition, I always tell people the best juicer is the one you will use. If a steep price tag is an excuse not to purchase a juicer, get an inexpensive one. Most of the popular kitchen appliance manufacturers offer models that use a spinning technique called "centrifugal juicers." While these types also spin air into the juice that may cause it to oxidize faster, it is still better than not drinking juices at all. The more expensive juicers are usually called "masticating juicers" and they tend to spin the juice slower and include more of the fibre, thereby increasing the amount of fibre, enzymes, vitamins, and minerals you'll get in your juice. Many of these juicers are multi-purpose, enabling you to make fruit or vegetable purées, baby food, fresh nut butters, and healthy frozen desserts. I use a Champion juicer that I've had for almost a decade for juicing, and I also like the Green Star juicer. You can also make "total juice" or "whole juice" in a high-powered blender, which I'll explain momentarily.

There are also juicers specifically suited for citrus fruits like lemons, limes, oranges, and grapefruits. Some are as basic as a wooden or ceramic reamer which is pushed into half of the fruit and turned while holding it over a pitcher or bowl. Other options are fully electric, involving pressing half of the citrus fruit down against a citrus reamer that spins. They range from plastic ones, which typically cost between $25 and $35 to stainless steel ones that typically cost around $150 to $175. I've used both electric and manual ones and prefer the inexpensive ceramic types that sit on the counter and have a handle to hold while you are pressing the citrus fruit with the other hand. Find one that has a small bowl that holds the juice for convenience. I then pour the juice through a strainer to remove any seeds that may have found their way into the juice.

Blender / Hand Blender / Personal Blender

My husband's birthday and my birthday are only a day apart, so about a decade ago we decided to buy a Vita-Mix blender as a joint birthday gift to ourselves. It was one of the best investments we've made for our health. Rarely does a day go by that we don't use it. More often, our Vita-Mix gets a workout at least several times a day to make soups, smoothies, frappés, total juices, almond milk, or some other healthy creation. A Vita-Mix is a high-powered blender that has the capacity to do much more than the stuff of other blenders. While its price tag tends to be in the $550 to $1250 range, depending on the model and the country of origin, it has so many uses that it makes a great addition to the life force diet. But, like I stated for juicers, it's not an essential item. If you have a standard blender, you can still make most, if not all, of the recipes that follow. And most blenders are under $50.

Personal-size blenders are also great. You can blend and serve in the same cup. Most of them come with multiple containers for different members of the household, along with caps to cover the blending container and take your smoothie on the go. I'll often put equal amounts of ingredients in two of the personal-size blender canisters, blend them into smoothies, add caps and take them as part of a picnic lunch or dinner with my husband, Curtis. We love being outdoors, so the personal blenders work well for us to take smoothies when we're hiking, biking, walking, or picnicking. But they work equally well if you don't have time for a sit-down breakfast, if you have an evening meeting, or the kids have to be rushed out the door for hockey, dance, piano lessons, or some other sport or lesson. They usually cost between $50 and $100, depending on the brand and number of accessories included. My sister gave us the Personal Blender brand as a gift a number of years ago, and we've used it regularly ever since to make under-a-minute fresh salad dressings, smoothies, and much more. It's an excellent addition to the life force diet.

Cooking Whole Grains

There are many delicious and nutritious whole grains that are simple to add to your diet. If you're pressed for time, choose the protein-packed, quick-cooking ancient grain quinoa. Top with vegetables for a nutritious and delicious meal in only 15 minutes. Quinoa is also free of gluten so it's a great choice for anyone needing to avoid gluten, including anyone suffering from celiac disease. Millet and brown and wild rice are also free of gluten. If you're suffering from mysterious health symptoms, digestive discomfort, or general aches and pains, choose only gluten-free grains. Many people find that an enzyme deficiency and a sensitivity to gluten may have been the culprit all along and that a break from gluten helps to rebuild their body and their health. Here's a cooking guide for preparing gluten-free whole grains to help you get started.

Cooking Guide for Whole Grains				
Grain	Amount of Grain	Amount of Water	Cooking Time in Minutes	Yield (Approximately)
Millet	1 cup	3 cups	30	4 cups
Quinoa	1 cup	2 cups	15	2¾ cups
Rice, brown	1 cup	2 cups	35–40	2½ cups
Rice, wild	1 cup	3 cups	50–60	3 to 4 cups

Sprout Out Loud

You'll need only a few basic supplies to get started sprouting. They include the following:

· Organic sprouting seeds, nuts, legumes, or grains
· Measuring spoons or cups
· Large wide-mouth jars
· Sprouting lids for jars (They are typically available in most health food stores. Alternatively, you can use cheesecloth and rubber bands over the top of the jars.)

Once you have everything ready, you're ready to start growing sprouts. You'll soon discover it is absolutely simple.

Step 1: Wash your hands thoroughly before handling seeds of any kind (seeds, nuts, legumes, or grains. For simplicity I'll be referring to any of these items as seeds in the following steps.)

Step 2: Remove any broken or discoloured seeds, stones, twigs, or hulls that may have found their way into your sprouting seeds.

Step 3: Place the seeds in the jar—only one type per jar unless you're using special sprouting seeds. Follow the amounts specified in the chart below. For the grains and beans be sure you're using large jars, since they will absorb water and grow substantially in size.

Step 4: Cover the seeds with pure water. If you are using a few tablespoons of seeds, cover with at least 1 cup of water. If you are using beans, nuts, or grains, use at least three times the water of the amount of seed. In other words, 1 cup of mung beans and 3 cups of water.

Step 5: Let soak for the specified amount of time, which is just a guideline. Often I'll start the soaking just before going to bed or first thing in the morning. The soak time typically ranges from 6 to 12 hours.

Step 6: Cover the jar with the sprouting lids or cheesecloth. If you're using cheesecloth, secure it over the top of the jar with a rubber band. Drain off the water.

Step 7: Rinse thoroughly and drain off the water again. Set upside down in a clean, cool spot in your kitchen area, preferably on a slight angle to allow excess water to drain off.

Step 8: Rinse the sprouts a few times a day (unless more is suggested below in the sprouting chart). Be sure to drain them well each time.

Step 9: (Optional): Once the sprouts have grown for the specified amount of time and are ready to be harvested, place them in a large bowl of cool water and stir them around to loosen hulls and skins from the seeds. They'll usually come to the top so you can remove them. Don't worry about removing every last one. This step helps prevent spoilage and encourages the sprouts to last longer. Drain sprouts well and store in the refrigerator for a week to 10 days.

TIP: To increase the mineral content of your sprouts, add a piece of kelp or other seaweed to the water while the seeds are soaking.

As you learned earlier, sprouts are packed with essential nutrients: vitamins, minerals, fibre, and loads of enzymes. While you can purchase them at your local grocery store or health food store, it is simple to grow your own. Growing your own is a great way to have a supply of gourmet varieties, ensure access to high-quality fresh foods year round if you live in a colder climate, or to readily add a serious amount of life force to your diet.

There are many ways to sprout, but I prefer using wide-mouthed Mason jars, with an inexpensive mesh, screw-on top available in most health food stores. You can also use sprouting trays, electric machines, or other systems. I've tried many kinds and always come back to the simple jar and sprout lid method, which just happens to be the most cost-effective method as well.

Simple Sprouting

Seed Type	Amount	Soaking Time	Sprouting Time	Approximate Yield	Sprout Length at Harvest	More Info
Aduki bean	½ cup	12 hours	3 to 5 days	4 cups	½" to 1½"	Best if rinsed a few times a day.
Alfalfa seed	3 Tbsp.	5 hours	3 to 6 days	3 to 4 cups	1" to 2"	To "green" the leaves, place in indirect sunlight on last day of sprouting.
Almond	1½ cups	8 to 10 hours	1 to 2 days	2 cups	Up to ⅛"	Most often eaten just soaked.
Amaranth grain	1 cup	3 to 5 hours	2 to 3 days	3 cups	Up to ¼"	Best if rinsed a few times a day.
Broccoli seed	2 Tbsp.	8 hours	3 to 4 days	2 cups	1" to 2"	Rinse a few times a day. Place in indirect sunlight last day of sprouting.
Buckwheat (hulled)	1 cup	6 hours	1 to 2 days	2 cups	⅓" to ½"	Best if rinsed every 30 minutes for the first few hours. Soak for no longer than 6 hours.

Continued on page 208

Simple Sprouting

Seed Type	Amount	Soaking Time	Sprouting Time	Approximate Yield	Sprout Length at Harvest	More Info
Cabbage seed	1 Tbsp.	4 to 6 hours	4 to 5 days	1½ cups	1" to 2"	Rinse 2 to 3 times a day, shaking vigorously.
Clover seed	3 Tbsp.	5 hours	4 to 6 days	3 to 4 cups	1" to 2"	"Green" leaves in indirect sunlight on last day.
Fenugreek seed	4 Tbsp.	6 hours	2 to 5 days	2½ to 3 cups	1"	Bitter if left to grow past 1".
Garbanzo bean (Chickpeas)	1 cup	12 to 48 hours	2 to 4 days	3 to 3½ cups	½" to 1"	To make them easier to digest, soak longer. Rinse often during sprouting process.
Kale seed	4 Tbsp.	4 to 6 hours	4 to 6 days	3 to 4 cups	¾" to 1"	Rinse 2 to 3 times a day.
Kamut grain	1 cup	12 hours	2 days	2 to 3 cups	¼ to 1/2"	Rinse often. Can use to make sprouted bread.

Lentil	¾ cup	8 hours	2 to 3 days	3 to 4 cups	½" to 1"	Rinse often. Be sure to remove broken or split lentils prior to soaking.
Mustard seed	3 Tbsp.	5 hours	3 to 5 days	3 cups	½" to 1½"	"Green" in indirect sun on last day of sprouting.
Oats (whole, hulled grain)	1 cup	8 hours	1 to 2 days	1 cup	Up to ⅛"	Rinse 3 times a day. Be sure to use whole, hulled grain that has not been steamed. Can be difficult to sprout.
Onion seed	1 Tbsp.	4 to 6 hours	4 to 5 days	1½ to 2 cups	1" to 2"	Rinse a few times a day.
Pinto bean	1 cup	12 hours	3 to 4 days	3 to 4 cups	½" to 1"	Rinse a few times a day minimum.
Pumpkin seed	1 cup	6 hours	1 to 2 days	1½ to 2 cups	Up to ⅛" sprout	It's fine to use them after soaking only. May not sprout.
Quinoa grain	1 cup	3 to 4 hours	2 to 3 days	3 cups	Up to ½"	Rinse thoroughly prior to soaking for best taste.

Continued on page 210

Continued from page 210

Simple Sprouting

Seed Type	Amount	Soaking Time	Sprouting Time	Approximate Yield	Sprout Length at Harvest	More Info
Radish seed	3 Tbsp.	6 hours	3 to 5 days	3 to 4 cups	¾" to 2"	Rinse thoroughly prior to soaking for best taste.
Rye grain	1 cup	6 to 8 hours	2 to 3 days	3 cups	½" to ¾"	Rinse a few times a day. Don't leave in overly warm environment.
Sesame seed (hulled)	1 cup	8 hours	Less than 1 day	2 cups	n/a	Will not sprout, but soaking increases nutrients and digestibility.
Spelt grain	1 cup	6 hours	1 to 2 days	2 cups	Up to ¼" sprouts	Replaces wheat in recipes.
Sunflower, hulled	1 cup	6 to 8 hours	Less than 1 day	2 cups	¼" to ½"	Skim off skins after soaking.

Teff seed	1 cup	3 to 4 hours	1 to 2 days	2½ to 3 cups	Up to ⅛"	Teff can be hard to sprout due to the seed's tiny size, which can escape even the finest mesh sprouting lid. Try cheesecloth held in place by an elastic over a glass jar.
Wheat grain	1 cup	8 to 10 hours	2 to 3 days	2 to 3 cups	¼" to ¾"	Use to make sprouted grain breads.

Occasionally you may find that a batch of seeds won't sprout. There are numerous possible reasons:

1. The seeds may have been old.
2. The seeds may have been irradiated prior to arriving on grocery store or health food store shelves.
3. The seeds may have been exposed to moisture during storage, either in your home or prior to purchasing them.
4. The seeds may have been exposed to excessive heat at home or prior to purchasing them. Oat groats and almonds are often heated to extend shelf life. Unfortunately the life force is destroyed during this process.
5. Refined or polished grains like rice, pearl barley, oats, or debittered quinoa will not sprout due to the refining process.
6. You may have soaked the seeds too long or too little. Refer back to the sprouting chart above.
7. Insects may have damaged the seeds.

Ancient Aztec peoples soaked nuts and seeds in water overnight before they drained them and dried them in the sun. They obviously experienced the digestive and health benefits of doing so, even if they didn't understand the modern science behind this practice. Nuts and seeds contain natural enzyme inhibitors like phytic acid, which, when eaten, can irritate digestion. A simple way to reduce the amount of these enzyme inhibitors is to soak nuts and seeds in pure, unchlorinated water overnight (or at least for a couple of hours), drain, and rinse. I usually soak nuts or seeds in the evening, drain them in the morning, and take a jar or bag for a quick and highly nutritious snack on the go. I encourage you to do the same. Most nuts will not sprout, but getting into the habit of soaking them before eating them not only makes them more digestible, it increases the nutrient and enzyme quantity in them.

Growing sprouts and soaking nuts are easy ways to add life force energy to your diet and therefore your body. While it is not necessary to grow your own sprouts, since they are readily available in many grocery and natural food stores, it is a great way to ensure a steady supply of nutrition and plentiful amounts of curative enzymes in your diet.

Spice Up Your Food

To season your food, choose fresh herbs like basil, oregano, parsley, or mint when you can find or grow them. It is also beneficial to keep dried herbs in your pantry for those times when it may be difficult to find fresh ones, or if you're preparing dinner in a hurry. Obviously fresh is superior both in flavour and in nutritional value, but dried, organic, non-irradiated spices are superior to simply salting your food. When you use salt, choose Celtic sea salt or Himalayan crystal salt. The former is greyish coloured while the latter has a peachy or orangey hue.

If you're not sure which spices to use in your food preparation, here's a quick reference chart to help you get started.

Spice Up Your Life	
Spice	**Uses**
Basil	A sweet and peppery aroma and flavour, basil is one of my favourite herbs. The fresh and dried versions have a distinctly different flavour. It can be chopped finely and added to soups, salads, tomato-based juices, salad dressings, sandwiches, wraps, and tomato sauces.
Celery Seed	Be sure to use celery seed, not celery salt. Celery seeds contain over 20 anti-pain and anti-inflammatory compounds and add a salty, celery flavour to soups, sauces, and stews.

Continued on page 214

Continued from page 213

Spice Up Your Life	
Spice	**Uses**
Chili Peppers	The colour and level of heat from fresh chili peppers varies greatly between varieties. Chili peppers not only add spiciness to foods, they also add fat-burning and anti-inflammatory healing properties to your favourite soups, stews, salad dressings, bean dishes, and Mexican and Latin American dishes.
Cilantro	Fresh cilantro looks like parsley but has a unique almost citrus flavour. It is an excellent addition to fresh salsa, soup, stew, curries, salads, tomato sauces, and noodle and vegetable dishes.
Cinnamon	Dried, powdered cinnamon has natural antibacterial properties, helps to balance and stabilize blood sugar levels, and burns excess fat. Plus, it just tastes great. It is excellent with apples, fruit dishes, curries, vegetables, and stews.
Ginger	Freshly grated, juiced, or chopped, ginger adds a warm, sweet kick to any food. It also adds tremendous anti-pain and anti-inflammatory action. If I ever feel pain or a headache coming on, I make a fresh juice with an inch or two-inch piece of fresh ginger juiced into it. You can also add fresh ginger to fruit dishes, breads, sweet potatoes, vegetables, curries, and Asian noodle dishes.
Oregano	Naturally anti-bacterial, anti-fungal, and antiviral, oregano also adds spice to your favourite Italian dish, including tomato sauces, salads, soups, and stews.
Parsley	Not just a garnish, fresh parsley is packed with minerals and other nutrients and deserves a place in your life force diet. It can be added to soup, pasta, sauces, salad dressings, salads, or as the main component of a yummy Middle Eastern salad called tabbouleh which also contains lemon juice, chopped tomatoes, and onions. I use cooked quinoa in place of the couscous for a healthier, protein-rich version of this traditional salad.

Rosemary	With its distinctive sweet and pine-like aroma and flavour, rosemary is a delicious addition to sweet potatoes, carrots, stews, sauces, marinades, salad dressings, or bread.
Sage	A pungent and aromatic spice, fresh sage can be added to tomato sauces, soups, stews, or made into a healthy Thanksgiving-style dressing using chopped whole grain bread, onions, green peppers, red peppers, celery, water or vegetable stock and some Celtic sea salt. Thrown into a casserole dish and baked at 350 F for an hour, this is a delicious dish any time of year.
Thyme	Pungent and slightly sweet, this herb is a great addition to tomato sauces, soups, stews, and beans.

Preparing food with fresh herbs and spices does not have to be intimidating. Try the recipes at the back of this book to help you get started and then start experimenting by following the suggestions in the above chart. Your palate and body will love you.

The Life Force Family

It may be tempting to push your new way of eating on everyone in your family. But remember, most people resist anything when it feels forced upon them. It is far better to start eliminating the 3 Ps from your family's diet by eliminating them from your home. By simply not making the 3 Ps available, your family is far less likely to eat them. These items are not foods and truly have no place in our diets, particularly not in the diets of growing children, whose brains and bodies are in critical formative stages. Exposing them to the myriad assortment of potentially toxic additives found in processed, packaged, and prepared foods poses a serious health threat. So start there. If people have to make an effort to get them, they are less likely to do so. Your family may insist on having processed, packaged, and prepared foods, but you don't need to purchase them if you're the one doing the grocery order.

Continue by choosing healthier alternatives like those outlined in Chapters 4 and 5 so they are readily available in your fridge and pantry.

Add a large dinner salad to every meal and make enough for all of your family members. By including items such as berries, avocados, orange slices, or dressings that include these items, salads have wide appeal—even to those who are not interested in being health-conscious. This simple step can spur an interest in eating regular salads that can have significant positive health implications.

By eating the life force diet, family members may be curious about the food choices you're making and may take an interest in learning why you're choosing them. Additionally, many will be interested in sampling some of your delicious-looking selections.

When I met my husband, he was a "meat-and-potatoes" man who rarely ventured into the territory of produce, other than the occasional iceberg lettuce salad, carrots, or broccoli florets. We frequently cooked separate meals. I recall our "spaghetti nights": We boiled two pots of water, one for his white spaghetti and one for my brown rice spaghetti noodles; he cooked a jar of tomato sauce while I diced onions, fresh tomatoes, red peppers, and basil for a homemade sauce. Over time, he noticed that my food simply smelled more aromatic and expressed interest in mixing a bit of my fresh tomato sauce with his jar of sauce. Once he realized how much better it tasted, he switched entirely to my fresh sauce and brown rice noodles. Now he eats the life force diet and loves it. He often tells people how much better the food tastes than the standard processed fare.

My sister and her husband have raised their two children on primarily Life Force Gold Foods since they were weaned off breast milk, and the results are phenomenal. They have rarely succumbed to any of the common childhood sickness or infections that are "going around." They are full of energy, without being hyperactive, and are active, and demonstrate mental capabilities far beyond their years.

What's more, they love the food. They choose fruit over candies and cakes any day. They crave salads and love a variety of tastes most children would snub. My sister even makes delicious enzyme-rich cakes for celebrations!

The Life Force Traveller

It's possible to have your frequent flyer miles and your life force diet too. With a little planning, you'll continue to reap the benefits of improved energy levels and delicious healthy foods. Here are some simple tips:

1. Bring your favourite digestive enzyme product to assist with digesting your food. Enzymes also help your body cope with foreign bacteria that your body may not be used to. Take one or two with every meal to help keep your digestion in tip-top shape.

2. Bring your favourite unsweetened green food supplement since they are packed with nutrients. If carefully selected, many green powders are also excellent sources of enzymes. Be sure to choose one that hasn't been heated during the manufacturing processes.

3. When travelling via plane or train, call in advance or when booking your ticket to check if a fruit plate or salad is available. Many airlines and rail companies offer these healthier options for a small charge when ordered alongside the ticket.

4. Bring pieces of fruit or pre-cut veggie sticks for car or bus trips should you have difficulty finding healthy options.

5. Choose a salad in restaurants without healthy food options. Simply ask for some lemon wedges and olive oil instead of dressing. Most restaurants are happy to accommodate this request. Most quality restaurants offer mixed green salads with leafy greens that actually resemble their name, but if the restaurants are calling iceberg lettuce a "green salad," just ask them to top it off with cucumber slices, green peppers, and tomatoes to try to increase its nutritional value.

6. Many international restaurants offer better options than those that offer only standard North American fare. Middle Eastern (Lebanese, Turkish, Persian, Egyptian), Greek, Mexican, and Asian (Japanese, Thai, and some Chinese) restaurants are often more likely to contain more vegetables, beans, and whole grains than the typical burger-and-fries options.

7. Raw nuts and seeds are excellent choices while travelling, since they offer a high amount of protein, essential fatty acids, and help keep blood sugar levels stable, thereby warding off cravings for unhealthy items.

8. Check the internet or local phone books to find out if there are any organic markets, health food stores, or health-focused restaurants in the areas where you'll be staying.

It takes some effort to eat the life force diet when you're on the road or in the skies, but the effort is definitely rewarded in the form of greater energy and vitality to stay healthier and ward off illness.

9

The Luscious Life Force Recipes

THIS chapter contains dozens of delicious life force recipes, including Peach Pineapple Ice Cream, Plumpaya Pudding, and many others. You'll love the delicious and decadent recipes in this chapter, many of which take only 10 minutes or less to prepare. Looking and feeling great never tasted so good!

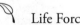 Life Force Gold Recipe

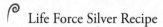 Life Force Silver Recipe

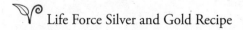 Life Force Silver and Gold Recipe

Breakfast

Eggless Scramble

Serves 4

This dish is loaded with nutrients and fibre from the vegetables and makes a great substitute for eggs to help keep your consumption of animal protein down. It is also high in lean protein and calcium. Turmeric, a spice commonly used in Indian cooking, is a great natural anti-inflammatory. You can also serve this recipe as a quick and delicious dinner.

8 oz. ·	firm tofu, crumbled
I tsp. ·	ground turmeric
I tsp. ·	Celtic sea salt
½ tsp. ·	ground cumin (optional)
4 ·	tomatoes, quartered
2 tbsp. ·	extra virgin olive oil
I ·	large onion, chopped
I ·	small sweet potato, chopped (optional)
2 ·	stalks celery, chopped
I ·	red bell pepper, chopped

1. In a bowl, combine tofu, turmeric, salt, and cumin; set aside.
2. In a blender or food processor, purée tomatoes; set aside.
3. In a large skillet, heat oil over medium-low heat, making sure it doesn't smoke. Sauté onion until softened. Add sweet potato (if using) and sauté until tender. Add celery and red pepper; sauté until tender. Add seasoned tofu and sauté until heated through. Stir in tomato purée, cover, and cook for 5 to 10 minutes, or until all ingredients are heated through and the flavours have blended.

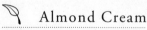 Mom's Apple Cinnamon Oats

Serves 1 to 2

My mom shared her quick and easy breakfast recipe which is great when you want something warm and packed with nutrition and flavour. It's loaded with vitamins, minerals, fibre, and enzymes.

⅓ cup · oatmeal
2 tbsp. · raisins
⅓ cup · water (boiling)
½ · apple, diced
1 tbsp. · ground flax
¼ tsp. · ground cinnamon
1 tbsp. · raw walnuts, chopped (optional)
· Almond Cream (recipe follows)

1. Place oats and raisins in a bowl and cover with the boiling water. Let sit for 2 minutes while dicing the apple.
2. Add the apple, cinnamon, and chopped walnuts (optional).
3. Top with Almond Cream and serve immediately.

Almond Cream

Serves 2

23 · raw almonds
½ cup · water
1 tsp. · maple syrup

1. Place all ingredients in a blender until smooth.
2. Pour over Mom's Apple Cinnamon Oats.

Jump-Start Breakfast Smoothie

Serves 1 to 2

Another one of my mom's excellent recipes, her Jump-Start Breakfast Smoothie is her breakfast of choice when she needs an instant morning jump-start instead of coffee. It's packed with life force enzymes, fibre, vitamins, minerals, and phytonutrients, all of which can help you get going in the morning. Don't be alarmed by the less-than-appetizing colour; this smoothie tastes great.

        1 · banana

     1 tbsp. · ground flaxseeds

     1 tbsp. · green powder (such as barley grass juice powder) or
                 1 cup of fresh spinach

      1 tsp. · coconut oil or flax oil

 1½ cups · frozen fruit (blueberries, strawberries, mangos, or green or
                purple grapes)

    2 cups · water (use more or less water, depending on preferred
                consistency)

Place all ingredients in a blender and blend until smooth. Drink immediately.

❧ Sprouted Grain Toast with Almond Butter
Serves 2

4 · slices sprouted grain bread, sliced and toasted (available at
most health food stores)
· Raw Almond Butter (see recipe below)
1 · banana or peach

1. Spread toast with Raw Almond Butter.
2. Top with banana or peach slices and serve immediately.

Option: Use fresh strawberries in place of bananas or peaches for a
real treat. Even finicky children love this recipe.

❧ Raw Almond Butter

Raw Almond Butter is an excellent source of fibre, calcium, magnesium, Omega 3 fatty acids, and medium-chain triglycerides—all
essential for building superb life force. When given the task of adding
more Omega 3s and medium-chain triglycerides to her diet, my mom
created this excellent recipe. It works well on toast, in sandwiches,
and on celery sticks or crackers.

3 cups · almonds
⅓ cup · coconut oil
½ cup · flax oil

1. Grind the almonds in a food processor until finely ground.
2. Add the coconut and flax oil. Process until smooth.
3. Store in a glass jar in the refrigerator for up to two weeks.

℮ Apple Pancakes

Serves 2

½ cup · whole grain kamut or spelt flour
1 tsp. · aluminum-free baking powder
½ tsp. · Celtic sea salt (finely ground)
1 cup · rice or almond milk
½ tsp. · cinnamon
1 · apple, sliced

1. Mix all ingredients (except apple slices) together.
2. Cook by scoopfuls in an oiled frying pan.
3. While the first side is cooking, push the apple slices into the batter. When golden brown, flip and cook the other side. Serve immediately.

Beverages

 Life Force Lemonade

Serves 4

Sipping on this delicious lemonade is a great way to escape the stresses of modern life. It instantly gives the feeling of a simpler, slower pace that is as refreshing to the psyche as drinking it is to the body. It naturally balances the body's biochemistry in favour of the more healing alkaline levels and helps cleanse the liver. What's more, unlike most sweetened lemonade, thanks to the naturally sweet herb stevia, this lemonade keeps blood sugar levels stable. It tastes so good even kids will love it.

> 5 · lemons
> 1 ½ tsp. · liquid stevia (approximately 90 drops) or more for a sweeter lemonade
> 6 cups · pure water
> · Ice cubes for serving
> · Fresh mint (optional, as garnish)

1. Juice the lemons using a wooden or ceramic lemon juicer (or use an electric citrus juicer if you have one). Pour the juice into a large pitcher.
2. Add the stevia and top with water. Stir to mix.
3. Pour over ice and add mint leaves (if using) to garnish. Serve.

Life Force Almond Milk

Serves 2 to 4

Make your own fresh and creamy almond milk to drink on its own or to use in baking or as a base in many of the following delicious fruit smoothies or baking recipes.

> 2 cups · purified alkaline water
> ½ cup · unsalted raw almonds
> 8 drops · liquid stevia

In a blender, blend water, almonds, and stevia until smooth. Strain, if desired.

TIP: Liquid stevia can be found in most health food stores.

 ## Water Berry Juice

Serves 2

Packed with the essential detox nutrient glutathione, watermelon supports your liver in eliminating toxic chemicals to which you may have been exposed. Combined with vitamin C–rich strawberries, this juice is a great cleanser and delicious too!

> 2 cups · watermelon (cubed)
> 1 cup · frozen strawberries

Blend watermelon and strawberries together until smooth. Serve.

Tropical Enzyme Smoothie

Makes 3 cups

This powerhouse of essential enzymes found in all the Life Force Gold Foods—pineapple, papaya, and banana—make this smoothie a great pick-me-up and super-healing drink. The combination of flavours makes it fantastic.

1½ cup · pineapple (chopped)
½ cup · papaya (chopped)
1 · banana
10 · ice cubes (or about 1 cup of ice)
½ cup · water

Blend all ingredients in a blender until smooth. Serve.

Option: Add 6 strawberries to this Tropical Enzyme Smoothie for a taste sensation.

 ## Green Goddess Juice

Makes 1½ to 2 cups

The tart and slightly sweet Granny Smith apple adds punch to the nutrient-packed celery and cucumber, making this lovely light green juice both yummy and healthy. The mint adds a great refreshing taste of summer.

4-inch · cucumber or piece of cucumber
6 · mint leaves
1 · Granny Smith apple
3 · stalks celery

Juice all ingredients together. Mix. Serve immediately.

Appetizers, Dips, and Spreads

 Southwestern Bruschetta

Serves 2 to 4

Here's a Mexican twist on an Italian favourite. I could eat this almost daily—it's that good. And it's easy to prepare for a snack, appetizer, or quick lunch.

> 4 to 6 · slices sprouted grain bread or yeast-free spelt or
>   brown rice bread
> 1 · clove garlic
>   · Life Force Avocado Salsa (see recipe on page 231)

1. Toast bread until fairly crisp.
2. Rub each slice with garlic.
3. Place on serving dishes and top with Life Force Avocado Salsa. Serve immediately.

Guacamole

Serves 2 to 4

Serve as a dip with Tortilla Chips (page 232) or carrot sticks, celery sticks, sliced red or green pepper, and broccoli or cauliflower florets. Or use as a spread on wraps and sandwiches. Eat soon after making, or the guacamole will discolour.

> 1 · avocado, peeled and pitted
> · Juice of ½ lime
> 1 tbsp. · organic cold-pressed flaxseed oil
> · Pinch Celtic sea salt

In a food processor, purée avocado, lime juice, flaxseed oil, and salt until smooth (or use a hand blender).

Variation: Garlic Guacamole

Add 1 clove of garlic with the avocado.

Michelle's Better Butter

Makes about 1 cup

Serve this soft, healthier butter substitute on warm Quick Spelt Bread (page 252) or any other bread recipe.

½ cup · organic extra virgin coconut oil
½ cup · organic cold-pressed flaxseed oil

1. In a small saucepan, over low heat, liquefy coconut oil. Immediately remove from heat and add flaxseed oil, stirring until well mixed.
2. Pour into a serving container and refrigerate until firm.

Make ahead: Store in an airtight container in the refrigerator for up to 6 months.

Variation: Michelle's Better Basil Butter

Immediately after adding the flaxseed oil, stir in a handful of chopped fresh basil.

Life Force Salsa

Serves 4 to 6

In only 5 to 10 minutes, you can enjoy this incredible fresh salsa, and it's so versatile! There are so many delicious uses for this yummy salsa. Below you'll find just a few ideas to help you get started.

1 ·	clove garlic
½ to 1 ·	small hot pepper, stem and seeds carefully removed (based on the level of heat desired)
1 ·	green onion, cut into 2-inch pieces
·	A small handful of fresh cilantro
3 ·	large tomatoes, cut in quarters
·	Juice of 1 lime
2 tsp. ·	ground psyllium hulls
½ tsp. ·	Celtic sea salt or Himalayan salt

1. In a food processor, process the garlic and hot pepper until finely minced.
2. Add green onions, cilantro, tomato wedges, lime juice, psyllium, and salt; pulse until coarsely chopped.
3. Serve with Life Force Tortilla Chips (see below), on celery sticks, on top of a plate of greens in place of dressing or on toasted sprouted grain bread for a quick and delicious appetizer.

Make ahead: Store in an airtight container in the refrigerator for up to 3 days.

Variation: Life Force Avocado Salsa

Add peeled, pitted, and cubed avocado just prior to serving. Toss gently to combine. The avocado cuts some of the heat and adds a creamy texture to the salsa.

℗ Life Force Tortilla Chips

Serves 2 to 4

In a matter of minutes you can enjoy healthy and delicious fresh tortilla chips.

I package · sprouted corn or sprouted grain tortillas
· Extra-virgin olive oil
· Celtic sea salt or Himalayan salt

1. Preheat oven to 350 degrees F.
2. Brush each tortilla with a small amount of olive oil and place in a single layer on baking sheets.
3. Sprinkle with salt and bake for 5 to 10 minutes or until lightly browned.
4. Break into chips and serve.
5. Serve with Life Force Salsa, as an accompaniment to chilli, salad, or soup. Or eat on their own instead of potato chips.

Make ahead: Wait until completely cooled and store in a jar or bag for use at a later time.

ꙮ Hummus

Serves 4

Hummus is a delicious Middle Eastern dip that has been part of the culture for thousands of years. It adds important fibre, vitamin C, iron, and calcium to your diet.

  2 cups · cooked chickpeas
        · Juice of 1 lemon
      1 · large clove garlic (or 2 small)
  ¼ cup · raw tahini (ground sesame seeds, also known as sesame
          butter)

1. In a food processor, purée all ingredients together until smooth.
2. Serve on sandwiches, as a dip for vegetable crudité, on wraps, or with Life Force Tortilla Chips (p. 232) or pita bread. I love it scooped up with celery as an appetizer or alongside a meal.

Make ahead: Store in an airtight container in the refrigerator for up to 1 week.

Soups and Stews

℘　　Veggie and Wild Rice Soup

Serves 6 to 8

3 tbsp. · olive oil
2 · medium onions, diced
2 · carrots, chopped
2 · potatoes, chopped
1 · small sweet potato, chopped
½ · small butternut squash, chopped
½ cup · wild rice
2 tsp. · Himalayan crystal or Celtic sea salt
10 cups · water
1 tsp. · dried basil
· Dash cayenne pepper

1. Sauté onions in olive oil over low to medium heat until lightly browned.
2. Put all ingredients in a large pot or slow cooker. Bring to a boil if stovetop cooking. Reduce heat and let simmer for 1 hour.
3. If using a slow cooker, cook on high for 6 to 8 hours.

ℓ Roasted Carrot Soup

Serves 2 to 4

6 · large carrots, chopped

2 tbsp. · extra virgin olive oil

2 · cloves garlic (whole)

½ tsp. · cumin

1 tsp. · Himalayan crystal or Celtic sea salt

· Dash cayenne pepper

3 - 4 cups · water, depending on preferred thickness

1. Sauté carrots in olive oil over low to medium heat until softened.
2. Add whole garlic cloves and continue sautéing until garlic is soft and carrots are lightly browned.
3. Place all ingredients in a blender and blend until smooth.
4. Heat and serve. If using a Vita-Mix blender, continue blending until soup is hot; then serve immediately.

℘ Miso Soup

Serves 2

This is the simplest soup I've ever tried. And it's a great way to add miso to your diet. Plus, it's warm and delicious, particularly on a cold winter evening. You can even enjoy this soup as a Japanese-style breakfast.

3 cups · water

3 tsp. · miso

1 · green onion, green end chopped

⅛ cup · silken tofu, cut into small cubes

1 tbsp. · arame or dulse seaweed, cut into fine strips (optional)

1. In a small pot, heat the water until boiling. Remove pot from heat.
2. Add the miso and whisk until the miso is well-blended.
3. Add the chopped green onion, diced silken tofu, and seaweed (optional). Let sit for a few minutes until seaweed is soft.
4. Stir and serve.

Savoury Lentil Stew

Serves 4 to 6

This hearty stew is perfect on a cold winter's night but is so delicious you'll want to eat it year round. It's packed with vitamin B1, potassium, iron, molybdenum, and other minerals. With 26 percent protein, lentil is the vegetable with the second highest level of protein (next to soybeans). What's more, only 1 cup of cooked lentils provides almost 90 percent of your daily requirement for folate and over 15 grams of fibre (that's a lot!). I've tried making this stew with French, green, and orange lentils—all with successful results, so use whatever kind you have on hand. And there's no need to worry about cooking them in advance. All you need are dried lentils. Enjoy.

1 tbsp. ·	extra virgin olive oil
1 ·	medium onion, diced
1½ cups ·	dried lentils
8 cups ·	water
1 ·	medium sweet potato, diced
1 ·	medium potato, diced
2 ·	stalks celery, chopped
1 tsp. ·	dried basil
1 tsp. ·	dried oregano
½ tsp. ·	dried thyme
1 tsp. ·	celery seeds
1½ tsp. ·	Himalayan or Celtic sea salt
·	Freshly ground black pepper to taste

1. In a large pot, heat the olive oil and sauté the onion until lightly browned.
2. Add the remaining ingredients and bring to a boil. Once the stew reaches boiling point, cover and simmer on low to medium heat for 1 hour or until the lentils are cooked.

Option: As a simple time-saver, combine all ingredients in a slow cooker in the morning. Cook on low heat for 6 to 8 hours. This delicious and hearty stew will be ready by the time you get home from work!

Celery and celery seeds (both of which are found in this Savoury Lentil Stew) contain over 20 anti-inflammatory and anti-pain compounds, according to America's best-known botanist, James Duke, PhD. Eat these foods regularly to maximize their pain-reducing powers!

What on Earth Is Rutabaga— and Why Would I Want to Eat It?

Rutabagas, or swedes, as they are often called in England, Wales, New Zealand, and Australia, are root vegetables with a light yellow and purplish hue. They offer delicious flavour to soup, stews, and curry dishes. They can also be cut and roasted, or steamed and mashed. They can also be grated and added to salads, particularly alongside carrots or apples. They are a good source of vitamin A, potassium, calcium, and magnesium. Because they are root veggies, they tend to be readily available even during winter months and are therefore inexpensive.

Salads and Salad Dressings

Tossing around Salad Ideas

If you avoid salads at any cost, thinking they consist only of iceberg lettuce and a couple of slices of starchy tomato topped with some chemical and sugar-laden bottled dressing, you will be happy to learn that life force salads are *so* much better than that. These excellent salads can be gourmet meals in themselves. I encourage you to make a large salad full of enzyme-rich Life Force Gold and Silver Foods the focal point of your meals at least once daily. Once you get started with this new habit, you'll see how easy and enjoyable it can be by simply being creative in your approach. I compiled the following list of ingredients to consider for salads and to prevent boredom. But this is just a guideline. There are many other possible ingredients that you can use to vary your salads from day to day:

Create a Gourmet Salad in Minutes	
Possible Salad Ingredients	
Apple slices	Celeriac or celery root
Apples (sliced or grated)	Chickpeas
Alfalfa sprouts	Chopped basil
Almond slivers (or chopped)	Chopped cilantro (coriander)
Avocado	Chopped mint
Beetroot (grated)	Chopped parsley
Blackberries	Clover sprouts
Blueberries	Cucumber
Boston lettuce	Edible flowers (such as nastur-
Broccoli sprouts	tiums, violas, or pansies)
Brown rice (cooked)	Endive
Carrots (julienned or grated)	Fenugreek sprouts
Celery	Broccoli (finely chopped)

Continued on page 240

Continued from page 239

Create a Gourmet Salad in Minutes
Possible Salad Ingredients

Fresh peas	Pine nuts
Grapefruit slices	Pinto beans
Grated cabbage	Pomegranate seeds
Grated carrots	Pumpkin seeds
Great Northern beans	Radicchio
Green onion	Radishes
Green peppers	Raspberries
Hazelnuts (chopped)	Red clover sprouts
Herbs (minced, such as basil,	Red peppers
thyme, oregano, garlic, and mint)	Romaine lettuce
Kidney beans	Seaweed (such as arame, nori,
Leaf lettuce	or wakame)
Lima beans	Sesame seeds
Mixed greens (mesclun)	Spinach
Mung bean sprouts	Strawberries
Mushrooms (raw or cooked)	Sunflower seeds
Olives	Sweet potato (grated)
Onion sprouts	Tomatoes
Orange slices	Watercress
Parsley	Wild rice (cooked)
Pea shoots	Yellow peppers
Peas (fresh)	

I'll often sauté or roast a few of my favourite foods like sweet potato wedges, red pepper slices, or onions (caramelized) and top a large plate of greens and raw veggies with these delicious ingredients. It's easy to add highly nutritious seaweed by soaking finely sliced seaweed like arame or wakame in water for 5 minutes to rehydrate, drain, and throw on top your other salad ingredients. Toss with one of my favourite dressings and have an instant delicious and gourmet salad.

The warmth of these ingredients offers a nice balance to the crunchy colder salad ingredients, particularly in the cold winter months.

Vegetable Crudités

You can add crunchy, enzyme-rich vegetables or fruit slices to a salad, or you can eat them on their own, or with a delicious dip. I try to keep a container packed with veggies that I've sliced or chopped into finger-foods for when I'm less than enthusiastic about preparing dinner or a snack. There are many veggies that are perfect for this purpose, including carrots or baby carrots, turnips, cucumbers, celery, radishes, green beans, cauliflower, tomato wedges, broccoli, and red, green, and yellow peppers. To keep them fresh after you've chopped them into matchsticks or wedges, store in a bowl of cold water with a squeeze of lemon and refrigerate.

Other Delectable Salad Additions

In addition to veggies, you can add fruit to your salads. Good options include apples, pineapples, tangerines, oranges, and pears. But you're really only limited by availability. Additionally, add marinated and cooked tempeh (fermented soybeans that has a naturally meaty taste); cooked organic chicken or beef; and grilled, baked, or steamed veggies.

Dressing Salads

Don't be intimidated by the thought of making your own salad dressings. They take only a couple of minutes, can be made in advance and stored in the refrigerator for a quick dressing when you need it, and are so much healthier than store-bought dressings.

Dressings can be made from cold-pressed oils such as extra virgin olive oil, walnut oil, flax oil, or a blend of healthy oils like Udo's Blend (available in most health food stores). You can add freshly squeezed lemon or lime juice (bottled concentrate does not count), apple cider vinegar (make sure it has a live culture in it, which means there will be some sediment in the bottom of the bottle), balsamic vinegar, or red or white wine vinegar. I have included some excellent salad dressing recipes to help you get started.

Typically, the ratio of lemon or vinegar to oil is one to three, making it easy to whip up your own creations. Then just add herbs, berries, or other ingredients to give your dressing even more flavour and nutrients. Shake all ingredients together in a covered jar or use a hand blender or personal blender to blend together for a thicker, smoother dressing. Most dressings will store for about a week in the fridge. I suggest keeping two or three on hand to add variety to your salads when you're pinched for time.

 Warm Black Bean Salad

Serves 2 to 4

> 1 tbsp. · extra virgin olive oil
> 1 · medium onion, diced
> 1 can · black beans, rinsed and drained
> ½ tsp. · oregano
> ½ tsp. · Himalayan crystal or Celtic sea salt
> 1 · tomato, chopped
> 1 · handful of fresh basil, minced

1. In a frying pan, sauté onion in the olive oil until slightly browned. Add the black beans, oregano, and salt, and continue sautéing for 1 to 2 minutes or until the black beans are heated through.
2. Remove from the heat and toss together with the tomato and basil. Serve immediately.

Provençal Salad Dressing

Serves 4

¼ cup · balsamic vinegar
¾ cup · extra virgin olive oil
1 tsp. · honey
1 tsp. · herbes de Provence
  · Dash Himalayan crystal or Celtic sea salt
  · Dash freshly ground black pepper

Mix all ingredients in a jar and shake or blend with a hand blender or personal blender.

Salade du Provence

1 bag · mixed greens
  · Handful alfalfa or clover sprouts
1 · avocado, pit and skin removed, sliced
1 cup · fresh blueberries

1. Toss mixed greens with Provençal Salad Dressing du Provence.
2. Place greens on serving plates. Top with sprouts, avocado, and blueberries. Serve immediately.

Life Force Salad

Serves 2 to 4

Don't let the strong-flavoured ingredients fool you; this salad is amazing. It's my favourite. Even if I'm not in the mood for salad, I can eat Life Force Salad. It earns the name because it is full of life force ingredients including greens, sprouts, garlic, ginger, citrus fruit juice, and more.

½ · onion, sliced finely (almost like shavings)
· Juice of ½ lemon or lime
· Dash Himalayan crystal or Celtic sea salt
2-inch · piece fresh ginger, julienned
1 · large or 2 small cloves fresh garlic, julienned
1 tbsp. · olive oil
1 · small package mixed greens
· Large handful or two of mung bean sprouts
1 · package of alfalfa, clover, or other sprout of your choice
(about 2 cups if you're growing your own sprouts)

1. Place onion slices in a small bowl. Add the juice of ½ lemon or lime and sprinkle the salt over it. Let sit for at least 5 minutes. This mellows the flavours of the onion. Reserve the liquid for the dressing (recipe below).
2. Heat the oil in a frying pan. Add the julienned ginger and garlic and cook until browned. Remove from the heat.
3. Place mixed greens on serving plates as a salad base. Top with bean sprouts and other sprouts being used.
4. Top with the onion slices and salad dressing.
5. Top with garlic and ginger crisps. Serve immediately.

Options: Add blood orange, orange, or grapefruit slices to salad. Top with avocado slices.

Life Force Salad Dressing

Serves 2 to 4

- Juice of · ½ grapefruit
- Juice of · ½ lemon or lime
- Juice of · ½ orange or mandarin
  - · Extra virgin olive oil
  - · Himalayan crystal or Celtic sea salt
  - · Freshly ground pepper

1. Put all ingredients in a jar (including reserved liquid from the onions) and shake until mixed.
2. Toss over salad ingredients.

৬৫ Thai Noodle Salad

Serves 4

Don't be alarmed by the lengthy ingredients list. You can assemble this delicious and incredibly fresh-tasting salad in 10 minutes. And if you're missing a couple of the salad ingredients, don't worry; just use what you have. After creating it the first time, I ate it every day for a week. It's that good! As an added bonus: You can make the dressing ahead and store it in the fridge for a week for a quick-and-easy lunch or dinner.

Salad Ingredients

- 1 · 8-oz. package of spelt, kamut, brown rice soba, udon, or spaghetti noodles
- ½ · package baby Romaine lettuce leaves
- 2 cups · mung bean sprouts
- 1 · carrot, grated
- 1 · red pepper, cut into 2-inch strips
- ½ cup · snow peas, cut in half lengthwise (optional)
- 1 · green onion, cut into diagonal pieces
- ½ cup · fresh cilantro, chopped
- ½ cup · raw, unsalted peanuts
- · Lime wedges to garnish

Dressing Ingredients

- ¼ cup · fresh cilantro
- ¼ cup · fresh mint
- ½ · green onion
- 1 · clove garlic
- 1-inch · piece fresh ginger
- 2 tbsp. · fresh lime juice
- 2 tbsp. · extra virgin olive oil
- ½ cup · almond milk
- ¾ tsp · salt
- · Dash cayenne

1. Cook the noodles in plenty of boiling salted water, drain, and set aside.
2. While the noodles are cooking, make the dressing. Place all dressing ingredients in a wide-mouth jar and blend with a hand-blender. Alternatively, blend all ingredients in a small blender or food processor. Set aside.
3. Place a base of lettuce on each plate. Add a handful of noodles to each. Then top with plenty of mung bean sprouts, carrots, red peppers, and snow peas. Sprinkle freshly chopped green onion, cilantro, and peanuts on top. Garnish with lime wedges.

Entrées and Side Dishes

Lentil Burgers

Makes approximately 8 burgers

1 · medium onion, diced
3 tbsp. · extra virgin olive oil
3 cups · cooked lentils, drained and rinsed
1 cup · quick-cooking oats
1 tsp. · Himalayan crystal or Celtic sea salt
½ tsp. · cumin
2 tbsp. · psyllium hulls/husks
· Freshly ground pepper to taste

1. In 1 tbsp. oil over low-medium heat, sauté chopped onion until lightly browned.
2. While the onion is cooking, mash lentils in a medium to large bowl using a potato masher. Add oats, salt, pepper, cumin, and psyllium hulls/husks. Mash together until mixed.
3. Add the cooked onions to the lentil mixture and stir together.
4. Form into burgers using your hands, being sure to press together firmly.
5. Heat remaining oil in the frying pan and cook burgers until browned on each side or about 5 minutes per side.

❧ The BLTP Sandwich

Serves 2

A healthier take on the traditional BLT, this sandwich is my husband's all-time favourite. It's so good you won't miss the bacon. Basil is the "B" in this sandwich. The "P" is for the roasted red pepper—a fantastic flavour combination!

>   4 · slices whole grain spelt or sprouted grain bread
> 2 tbsp. · extra virgin olive oil
>   1 · red pepper
>   1 · small package fresh basil
>   6 · whole peppercorns or freshly ground black pepper to taste
>   ¼ tsp. · Himalayan crystal or Celtic sea salt
>   1 · clove garlic, peeled
>   1 · tomato, sliced
>   · Lettuce

1. Heat a grill.
2. Brush one side of each slice of bread with olive oil.
3. Cut the red pepper into 4 large pieces and brush with a small amount of olive oil. Grill on both sides on the grill.
4. With a mortar and pestle (or food processor if you prefer) combine 1 tbsp. olive oil, basil, peppercorns, and sea salt until all ingredients form a fine paste.
5. Grill the bread on both sides and remove from the heat when finished.
6. Rub the fresh garlic clove over the dry side of each slice of grilled bread.
7. Spread the basil mix on one side of 2 slices of bread
8. Place the grilled red pepper on top of the basil mix. Add the tomato slice, lettuce, and other slice of grilled bread and serve.

℣ Pineapple Basil Rice

Serves 2 to 4

Okay, I must confess: I'm not a big fan of brown rice. I eat almost any other healthy food, but brown rice doesn't do much for me. So I'm always trying to come up with unique and delicious ways to prepare it to get it into my diet. I'd eat Pineapple Basil Rice every day and absolutely love it even though it is made with brown rice. It's so good even brown-rice haters will love it.

> 1 cup · brown rice
> 2 cups · water
> 2 tbsp. · coconut oil
> 1 · large handful fresh basil leaves
> ¾ cup · finely diced fresh pineapple
> ½ tsp. · Himalayan crystal or Celtic sea salt

1. Combine the rice, water, and 1 tbsp. of coconut oil in a small- to medium-size pot. Bring to a boil. Once the water begins to boil, immediately reduce heat to low and let simmer for 45 to 50 minutes or until all the water has been absorbed.
2. In a medium to large bowl, toss together the cooked rice, remaining coconut oil, basil, pineapple, and salt until combined. Serve immediately.

℘ Pasta Alfredo with Asparagus

Serves 2 to 4

1 pkg.. · brown rice pasta
12 stalk. · asparagus, ends trimmed and cut into 1-inch pieces

Bring a large pot of water to boil. Add the pasta and cook according to the package directions. While the pasta is cooking, sauté the asparagus in a few tablespoons of water in a large covered frying pan. Cook until tender but not mushy. Set aside in a small bowl. Drain the pasta when it has finished cooking and set aside. In the frying pan, prepare the Alfredo Sauce as indicated below. Once thickened add the pasta and asparagus to the frying pan and toss to coat.

Alfredo Sauce

1 tbsp. · extra virgin olive oil
1 · clove fresh garlic, minced
1 tbsp. · brown rice flour
1 cup · almond milk (unsweetened)
½ tsp. · Himalayan crystal or Celtic sea salt
· Freshly ground black pepper to taste

Heat oil in a pan over medium heat. Add garlic and sauté for 1 minute or until lightly golden. Add rice flour and stir to combine until lightly browned. Add almond milk, salt, and pepper; mix until combined and mixture thickens. Stir cooked pasta into sauce immediately. Toss and serve immediately.

℘ Quick Spelt Bread

Serves 10 to 12

> 1¾ cup · whole-grain spelt flour
> ½ cup · multigrain cereal or whole oats
> 1½ tsp. · baking powder (make sure it is "aluminum-free")
> 2 tbsp. · water
> 1¼ cup · rice or almond milk
> 2 tbsp. · honey
> ½ cup · canola or coconut oil (If using canola oil, choose cold-pressed organic preferably.)
> 2 tbsp. · ground flaxseeds (or grind your own in a coffee grinder)

1. Mix the flour, cereal, and baking powder together in a food processor or mixer.
2. In a separate bowl, whisk liquid ingredients together with the ground flaxseeds.
3. Slowly pour the wet ingredients into the dry ingredients. Stir until mixed.
4. Pour into a greased loaf pan and bake at 350 degrees F for 50 to 55 minutes.
5. Let sit for 5 to 10 minutes before removing from the loaf pan and serving.

❧ Grilled Salmon with Salsa Violetta

Serves 2

I could eat this amazing dish regularly. The garam masala dry rub is a wonderful contrast against the fresh, sweet taste of the Salsa Violetta.

2 · salmon fillets or 2 salmon steaks
1 tsp. · garam masala powder
¼ tsp. · Himalayan crystal salt

1. Rub the garam masala and salt into the top side of the salmon fillets (opposite the skin side).
2. Grill for 3 minutes skin side down if using fillets or 5 minutes if using steaks. Flip.
3. Cook for 3 minutes if using fillets or 5 minutes if using steaks.
4. Serve with Salsa Violetta (see recipe below).

Salsa Violetta

1 · black plum
½ cup · fresh purple grapes
· Small handful of fresh cilantro
⅓ cup · fresh or frozen blueberries
· Dash Himalayan crystal or Celtic sea salt
· Splash white wine vinegar
½ tsp. · honey

1. Remove the pit from the plum and dice into small cubes. Place in a small bowl.
2. Cut the purple grapes into quarters. Add to the diced plums.
3. Chop the cilantro and add to the plums and grapes.
4. Add the remaining ingredients to the bowl and toss to mix together.
5. Spoon over grilled salmon.

℗ Green Bean Ragout

Serves 2 to 4

1 tbsp. ·	extra virgin olive oil
2 ·	cloves fresh garlic, minced or pressed
3 ·	tomatoes (medium-sized), chopped
1 ·	small package of fresh green beans, ends removed (approximately 1½ cups). If unavailable use frozen.
1 ·	small zucchini, cut in large chunks
⅛ tsp. ·	Himalayan crystal or Celtic sea salt to taste
·	Freshly ground black pepper to taste

1. Sauté garlic in olive oil until slightly golden (1 to 2 minutes).
2. Add chopped tomatoes, green beans, zucchini, salt, and pepper, and cover with a lid. Allow to simmer over low to medium heat for 10 to 15 minutes or until veggies are cooked but not mushy.

Desserts

 ## Strawberry-Blueberry Pudding

Serves 2

This is a quick and easy way to satisfy a sweet tooth. From fridge to fantastic in under 5 minutes!

        1 · avocado, peeled and pitted
          · Juice of ½ lemon
    ½ cup · frozen blueberries
    ½ cup · fresh strawberries, washed and hulled

Place all ingredients in a food processor and process until smooth. Alternately, use a hand blender. Serve immediately.

 ## Brazilian Vanilla Ice Cream

Serves 2 to 4

This is the fastest, easiest, and most nutritious ice cream you can make. What's more, not only does it taste great, you don't need an ice cream machine to make this yummy treat. As long as you have a fairly high-powered blender, you can enjoy this soft-serve dessert.

    ⅔ cup · raw, unsalted Brazil nuts
    ⅔ cup · fresh medjool dates, pitted (or about 8 to 10 dates, de-
            pending on preferred sweetness)
    ½ cup · water
    2 tsp. · pure vanilla extract
      20 · medium-sized ice cubes

1. Blend the Brazil nuts, dates, water, and vanilla together until smooth.
2. Add the ice cubes and blend until smooth. Serve immediately.

Chocolate Truffles

Makes 12 truffles

Forget the double boilers, thermometer, and delicate techniques required to make traditional truffles. These delectable bites take minimal effort and can be made in under 15 minutes. They satisfy even the worst chocolate cravings, yet are packed with calcium, magnesium, fibre, and life force too!

⅔ cup · raw almonds
6 · fresh medjool dates, pitted
2 tsp. · maple syrup
2 tbsp. · cocoa and more to coat truffles in

1. Grind almonds in a food processor. Once finely ground, add dates, maple syrup and cocoa and process until smooth.
2. Take a large teaspoonful of the almond chocolate mixture and roll into a ball between your palms.
3. Roll in cocoa to coat.
4. Continue with steps 2 and 3 until all almond chocolate mixture is used.

Plumpaya Pudding

Serves 2 to 4

The key to the creamy texture and sweet taste of Plumpaya Pudding is in using fruit that is really ripe. I like using black plums since they are really sweet. Papayas are ripe when their skin turns quite yellow and the flesh yields slightly to touch. These fruits offer an excellent combination of delicious taste and excellent nutrition.

> 4 · ripe plums, pits removed, skin left on
> ½ · small papaya, peeled and seeded (or approximately
>   1 cup cubed papaya)
> 1 tsp. · unpasteurized honey

1. Mix all ingredients together in a blender until smooth.
2. Chill and serve.

 ## Peach Pineapple Ice Cream

Serves 2 to 4

This is one of the most delicious ice creams I've ever tasted. It's so good no one will know it's healthy. Yet it couldn't be easier to make. It takes about 5 minutes, plus a couple of hours' freezing time. You'll enjoy plentiful amounts of pain-relieving enzymes plus a blast of beta carotene for strong eyes and healthy skin.

> 2 cups · pineapple, outer skin and core removed and cut into cubes
> 2 · peaches, skins left on
> 1 tsp. · unpasteurized honey

1. Mix all ingredients together in a blender until smooth.
2. Pour into empty ice cube trays and place in the freezer for 2 to 3 hours, depending on the size of the ice cubes.
3. Serve as is or whip in a food processor just prior to serving.

Strawberry Chocolate Royale

Serves 2 to 4

This sinfully delicious dessert is perfect for a romantic evening or to satisfy a chocolate craving. It can be whipped up in a matter of minutes.

6–10 · strawberries
1 · banana
1 · large avocado
3 tbsp. · organic cocoa powder
2 tbsp. · pure maple syrup

1. Wash the strawberries. Remove hulls and cut into slices. Peel the banana and cut into slices. Set aside.
2. Cut the avocado in half lengthwise and remove pit. Scoop the flesh into a medium-sized bowl.
3. Add the cocoa powder and maple syrup. Using a hand blender, mash the avocado, cocoa, and maple syrup together until the cocoa powder is integrated. Blend until smooth.
4. To serve, place a scoop of the chocolate-avocado mixture into the bottom of two wine glasses. Add a layer of banana slices. Add a layer of strawberry slices. Continue layering the chocolate mixture with the bananas and strawberries until all ingredients are used.

TIP: This dessert is best when served immediately.

Strawberry Gelato

Serves 4

This delicious treat has a way of disappearing in a hurry. Once you've tasted it, you'll completely understand how it makes its disappearing act. In addition to being packed with life force enzymes, it's also a snap to make. Plus, you can have this delicious Italian-style soft ice cream in only a few minutes.

1 ½ cups · fresh pineapple, cut in cubes
2 cups · frozen strawberries
1 cup · frozen cranberries
1 cup · water

Blend all ingredients in a blender. If your blender has a plunger attachment you can use it to coax the ingredients to blend smoothly. Serve immediately.

Cranberry Creations

Most people know of cranberries' reputation for maintaining a healthy urinary tract, but few people know that it may also improve gastrointestinal and oral health (possibly protecting against tooth decay), help protect against kidney stones, balance cholesterol levels, assist in stroke recovery, and may even help prevent cancer. Cranberries contain the natural substance hippuric acid and other compounds that reduce the ability of the harmful bacteria *E. coli* to adhere to the walls of the urinary tract. The natural proanthocyanidins found in cranberries change the structure of *E. coli* in the body and even prevent these potentially harmful bacteria from communicating. Cranberries are also proving effective as anti-virals as well and may even be effective against herpes simplex 2. Research conducted at the University of Scranton, Pennsylvania, found that cranberries contain five times the antioxidants of broccoli. That's a nutritional powerhouse by anyone's standards. Now you can enjoy health-creating cranberries in delicious Strawberry Gelato.

Endnotes

Introduction

1. "Diet," http://www.thefreedictionary.com/diet.

CHAPTER 1

1. "How Many Animal Cells Can Fit on the Head of a Pin?" http://answers. yahoo.com/question/index?qid=20061003133913AAkNbgP.

2. Bill Bryson, *A Short History of Nearly Everything* (New York: Broadway Books), p. 377.

3. Peter Fraser et al. *Decoding the Human Body-Field* (Rochester, VT: Healing Arts Press, 2008).

4. Fraser et al. *Decoding the Human Body-Field.*

5. Bernard Jensen, PhD, *Dr. Jensen's Guide to Body Chemistry and Nutrition* (Columbus, OH: McGraw-Hill, 2000), p. xi.

6. Carla Golden, "New Bones in Ninety Days," http://goldencarla.typepad.com/ carla_goldens_get_healthi/2008/05/new-bones-in-ni.html.

CHAPTER 2

1. Jack Challem, *Feed Your Genes Right* (Hoboken, NJ: John Wiley & Sons, Inc., 2005), p. x.

2. Ibid., p. xiv.

3. Vincent E. Pernell, MD, "Essential Fatty Acids," http://www.drpernell.com/ essential_fatty_acids.htm.

4. Ibid.

5. "Minerals," http://www.essense-of-life.com/moreinfo/minerals/minerals.htm.

CHAPTER 3

1. Edward Howell, *Enzyme Nutrition* (Wayne, NJ: Avery Publishing, 1985).

2. Brian R. Clement, *Living Foods for Optimum Health* (Roseville, CA: Prima Health, 1998), p. 39.

3. Ibid., p. 39.

4. Ibid., p. 36.

5. Dr. Anthony J. Cichoke, *Enzymes & Enzyme Therapy* (Los Angeles, CA: Keats Publishing, 2000), p. 163.

6. "Worldwide AIDS & HIV Statistics," http://www.avert.org/worldstats.htm.

7. Cichoke, *Enzymes & Enzyme Therapy*, p. 163.

8. Kathleen Willcox and Helen Matatov, "The enzyme cure," *First for Women*, July 30, 2007, pp. 30–33.

9. Ibid., pp. 30–33.

10. Howell, *Enzyme Nutrition*, pp. 64–67.

11. Tom Bohager, *Everything You Need to Know About Enzymes* (Austin, TX: Greenleaf Book Group Press, 2008).

12. A. V. Everitt, et al., "Life extension by calorie restriction in humans," *Annals of the New York Academy of Sciences*, October 2007, 1114: 428–33.

13. Cichoke, *Enzymes & Enzyme Therapy*, p. 75.

14. Ibid., p. 75.

15. Ibid., p. 78

CHAPTER 4

1. Mikkel Hindhede, "The Effect of Food Restrictions During War on Mortality in Copenhagen," *Journal of the American Medical Association* 74,6 (1920): p. 381.

2. Magalie Lenoir, et al., "Intense Sweetness Surpasses Cocaine Reward" *PLoS ONE* (Bordeaux, France: Université Bordeaux, August 1, 2007) http://www.plosone.org/article/fetchArticle.action?articleURI=info%3Adoi%2F10.1371%2Fjournal.pone.0000698.

3. Lynn Melcombe, *The Health Hazards of Sugar* (Vancouver: Alive Books, 2001), p. 30.

4. Joseph Mercola, M.D. "Sweet Deception," http://products.mercola.com/sweet-deception/.

5. Michelle Schoffro Cook, *The Ultimate pH Solution* (Toronto: HarperCollins Publishers Ltd., 2008), p. 13.

6. "Ten Steps to a Healthy 1998," http://www.cspinet.org/nah/janfeb98.htm.

7. "Importance of Detoxification," Informational Brochure. (Advanced Nutrition Publications, Inc., 1994).

8. Patricia Fitzgerald, *The Detox Solution* (Santa Monica, CA: Illumination Press, 2001), p. 70.

9. Michelle Schoffro Cook, *The 4-Week Ultimate Body Detox Plan*, (Hoboken, NJ: John Wiley & Sons, Inc., 2006), p. 27.

10. Michelle Schoffro Cook, *The Brain Wash*, (Toronto: John Wiley & Sons Canada, Ltd., 2007) p. 75.

11. Patricia Fitzgerald, *The Detox Solution*. (Santa Monica, CA: Illumination Press, 2001), p. 73.

12. K. Singh, et al., "Studies on the Effect of Monosodium Glutamate (MSG) Administration on the Activity of Xanthine Oxidase, Superoxide Dismutase and Catalase in Hepatic Tissue of Adult Male Mice." *Indian Journal of Clinical Biochemistry*. Vol. 17, No. 1, January 2002, pp. 29–33.

13. Mercola, "12 Additives to Avoid," http://articles.mercola.com/sites/articles/archive/2008/06/24/12-food-additives-to-avoid.aspx?source=nl.

14. Schoffro Cook, *The Ultimate pH Solution*, p. 10.

15. Carly Weeks. "Ban Urged on Food Dyes Linked to Behavioural Problems." *Globe and Mail*, June 4, 2008. http://www.theglobeandmail.com/servlet/story/RTGAM.20080604.wlcolour04/BNStory/specialScienceandHealth/home.

16. Mercola, "12 Additives to Avoid."

17. Ibid.

18. Ibid.

19. Ibid.

20. Joseph Mercola, M.D. "Health Risks of Genetically Modified Foods," http://articles.mercola.com/sites/articles/archive/2000/12/03/ge-food-part-one.aspx.

21. Joseph Mercola, M.D. "GM Crops Can Produce Pesticides Inside Your Intestines," http://v.mercola.com/blogs/public_blog/gm-crops-can-produce-herbicide-inside-your-intestines-15869.aspx.

CHAPTER 5

1. Brenda Kearns, "Superfood Discovery," *First*, July 9, 2008, pp. 30–33.

2. "Phytonutrients: Prevention in a Plant – AOL Body," http://body.aol.com/medical-myths/phytonutrients-prevention-in-a-plant.

3. Ibid.

4. Brenda Kearns, "Superfood discovery," *First*, July 9, 2008, pp. 30–33.

5. Hatherhill, *The Brain Gate: The Little-Known Doorway That Lets Nutrients in and Keeps Toxic Agents Out*, p. 89.

6. Kearns, "Superfood Discovery," pp. 30–33.

7. Kearns, "Superfood Discovery," pp. 30–33.

8. Earl Mindell, PhD. *Earl Mindell's Food as Medicine* (New York, NY: Pocket Books, 2002), p. 109.

9. Ibid., p. 100.

10. Ibid., p. 111.

11. World's Healthiest Foods "Pinto Beans," http://whfoods.org/genpage.php?tname=foodspice&dbid=89#descr.

12. World's Healthiest Foods, "Bell Peppers," http://whfoods.org/genpage.php?tname=foodspice&dbid=50#descr.

CHAPTER 6

1. Wikipedia, "Sprouting," October 8, 2008, http://en.wikipedia.org/wiki/Sprouting.

2. Ibid.

3. Ibid.

4. Ibid.

5. Ibid.

6. Ibid.

7. Virginia Worthington, "Nutritional Quality of Organic Versus Conventional Fruits, Vegetables, and Grains," *The Journal of Alternative and Complementary Medicine*, Vol. 7, No. 2, 2001, pp. 161–173.

8. *The Organic Newsline* from organicTS.com, Vol. 3, Issue 3, September 2002.

9. Michelle Schoffro Cook, *Healing Injuries the Natural Way*, (Victoria, BC: Your Health Press, 2004).

10. "Lemons/Limes," George Mateljan Foundation, http://www.whfoods.com/genpage.php?tname=foodspice&dbid=27.

11. University of California at Berkeley, "News Release: February 21, 1996," http://berkeley.edu/news/media/releases/96legacy/releases.96/14316.html.

12. Amanda Ursell, *Complete Guide to Healing Foods* (London: Dorling Kindersley, 2000).

13. Steven G. Pratt, MD, and Kathy Matthews, *SuperFoods Rx* (New York, NY: HarperCollins, 2004).

14. Natalie Savona, *Wonderfoods* (London, Quadrille Publishing Limited, 2006).

15. Earl Mindell, PhD. *Earl Mindell's Food as Medicine* (New York, NY: Simon & Schuster, 1994).

CHAPTER 7

1. Tom Bohager, *Everything You Need to Know about Enzymes* (Austin, TX: Greenleaf Book Group Press, 2008).

2. "The no-cost way to erase fatigue forever!" *Woman's World*, May 12, 2008, p. 5.

Index

B